50 Reasons to be Happy

It's Not Always Bad News

By Jack Huber

Books by Jack Huber:

Non-Fiction:
50 Reasons to be Happy
RV Life Happens
A Poet's Primer- A Guide to Poetic Forms

Poetry:
Trappings of the Years
A Troupe in Masquerade
An Eerie Calm Before the Night
A Splendid Alternative
Aspects Long Forgotten
The Dilettante's Garden

Pat Ruger Mystery Series:
Pat Ruger: For Hire
Pat Ruger: Caribbean Shuffle
Pat Ruger: Native Species
Pat Ruger: Children's Reprise
Pat Ruger: Seattle Reign
Pat Ruger: Oblivion Highway
Pat Ruger: Music City Mayhem

E-Motion Publishing
First Printing, April 2021

Table of Contents

Foreward

Back in January, 2020, before the public knew the pandemic was coming, there was a disturbing amount of bad news in all media outlets. My wife, Nadyne, and I are retired, full-time RV'ers, living and moving around the country in our 31-foot fifth wheel and one-ton diesel pickup. It seemed like, no matter where we were, the news was negative. There were renewed tensions between the U.S. and Iran after the top Iranian military officer and known terror strategist was assassinated by American forces. More and more schools and shopping centers were targeted by active shooters. A major federal website was hacked by foreign operatives. Trump was gearing up for his re-election campaign, and the U.S. announced its very first case of COVID-19.

I decided that our life was not as bad as it seemed and that I could find a few things to write about, things that actually made us happy. I started a blog and posted a few articles about small, possibly forgotten, sources of happiness. I had some immediate positive feedback from readers and I continued to add new topics. The theme of the blog was that happiness can be fleeting unless it is pointed out and appreciated. We aren't religious or even spiritual people, but there are benefits to acknowledging there are things to be happy about and being thankful for them.

The tag line I use is "It's not always bad news." I keep that in mind when determining new topics and in describing reasons to be happy. After dozens of articles, I decided to publish the first 50 topics in a book. The list is in no particular order, and, in fact, many are placed just in the order I thought of them. None are political, as far as I can describe happiness in a nonpartisan way. Also, keep in mind that this is my personal list — you may have other subjects or items you would rank before mine — and that's OK. It's also not an exhaustive list — baseball is included but not football, golf or tennis — so I may well have enough topics for a sequel in a few months.

Here are a few words from my good friend and fellow author, Gerri Almand, who wrote *The Reluctant RV Wife* and *Home is Where the RV Is*, published by Brown Posey Press:

In February 2020 my husband and I attended an RVillage Rally in Live Oak, Florida, and camped next door to Jack and Nadyne Huber. Our obvious first connection with them was through RVing. Jack and Nadyne became our most trusted mentors for the transition from part-time to full-time nomadism.

Writing was the second connection. I found myself in awe of Jack's talent, productivity, and success. He quickly became my go-to source for writing and marketing strategies during a pandemic that left us running for our lives.

I am proud to introduce Jack's latest work. This anthology of "50 Reasons to be Happy," coming after a year-long cloud of COVID-19 stresses, brightens the gloom and reminds us that the world contains wondrous beauty and possibility. The diversity of Jack's topics is but a small indication of his breadth of knowledge and variety of interests. Thank you, Jack, for brightening my day with these cameos. I feel confident this will become a beloved collection for your readers.

You can find Gerri and her books on Amazon at *amazon.com/Gerri-Almand/e/B07W8679TS*

1. Food

If you ever wonder if food makes people happy, all you need to do is walk through a campground on a Saturday morning and let the smell of sizzling bacon and hot coffee fill your senses. OK, maybe not if you are a veggie person, but I'm sure you understand. Food is behind only air and water in our day-to-day survival needs and we as a species have made the most of it (with the help of fire, of course).

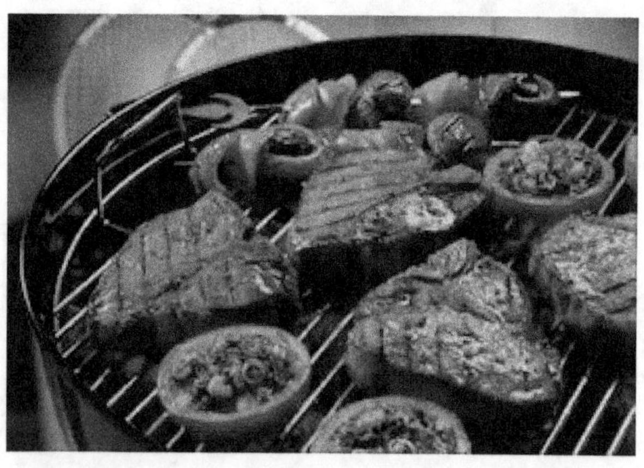

What about food makes me happy? As a carnivore, I am optimistic for the brilliant future of meat production. Not only are more humane and natural processes being put in place, but I am very much looking forward to mass-produced lab-grown meat. When they perfect the texture, taste and consistency, which isn't too far off, it could drastically scale back raising and killing livestock.

Second, have you ever stopped by a restaurant and ordered a dish that ended up being very similar to something your mother used to make? I have had the occasion to experience this and have enjoyed the memories immensely. It seems that sound, smell and taste can take you right back to a point in your past, no matter how remote, and food encompasses two of those.

Food can be a comfort, no doubt. Sometimes this can become a problem, but most of the time it just lets you deal with life. There's a reason men become grill masters and women spend the entire day making spaghetti. Before you complain about stereotypes, I concur. There are women who barbecue and men who make killer pasta. But the stereotype about those foods being comforting can't be denied.

Let's not forget the importance of a balanced diet. What comprises a balanced diet has continually changed with the science, but the old food pyramid was taught for generations. Per Wikipedia, "A food pyramid is a representation of the optimal number of servings to be eaten each day from each of the basic food groups. The first pyramid was published in Sweden in 1974. The 1992 pyramid introduced by the United States Department of Agriculture (USDA) was called the 'Food Guide Pyramid' or 'Eating Right Pyramid' ...

The pyramid was divided into basic foods at the base, including milk, cheese, margarine, bread, cereals and potato; a large section of supplemental vegetables and fruit; and an apex of supplemental meat, fish and egg. "

Last, I'll say that there is little in life that is more satisfying as enjoying one of the best steaks, fried chicken, corned beef and cabbage, grande burritos, or whatever you fancy as your favorite meal, that you've ever had. I'll grant you that it doesn't happen often enough, but when it does, bliss.

Growing up in my Southern California neighborhood, there were seven different fruit trees we all had access to. We had lemons, avocados and plums, two doors down were loquats and kumquats, one more house away was a green apple tree, and across the street had peaches, though I didn't like them. Most of these trees produced fruit year-round, but the summers were especially fun — having such variety of fresh fruit every day were good memories.

==================

I'll leave this topic with a quote from Robert Frost: *"Laughter is brightest where food is best."*

2. Driving

There's a lot about driving people dislike, i.e., traffic jams, accidents, tickets, and more. They don't call it "road rage" for nothing. But, it's not all bad.

In fact, I've LOVED driving since I first sat behind the wheel. My dad owned a gas station and I started working summers there when I was twelve. The service station was also a U-Haul dealer and by the time I was 14, I was moving those big U-Haul trucks around the lot and getting them parked. I bought my first car when I turned 16 and got my license. It was a 1962 white Econoline pickup, and I drove that truck with glee for a couple of years before buying a muscle car when I was nearly 18.

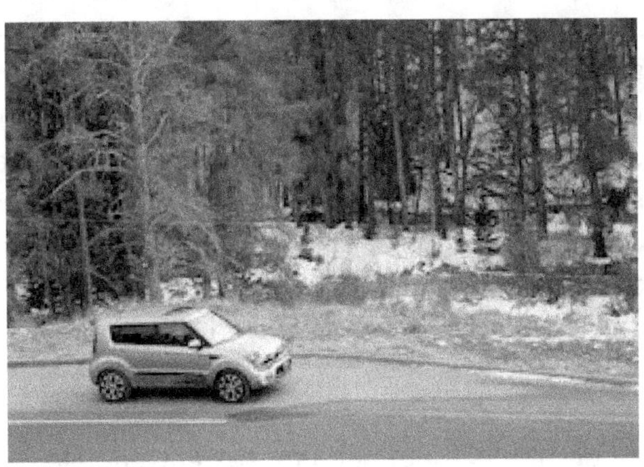

My 1970 Plymouth Duster was my "coming-of-age" car. Having pegged out the speedometer at 120 mph numerous times, I can only guess what its top speed was. I was young and invincible, and my driving showed it. However, starting a family made me much more aware of the dangers of speed and I reined myself in. By the time I was into my 20s, that Duster had carried us to San Francisco, Sequoia and Yosemite National Parks, Modesto and Merced in the Big Valley, and Joshua Tree National Forest and even Ensenada, Mexico, and all points in between.

I was a true explorer and have been ever since. No wonder we moved into our RV the moment we could. Since then, the sights have been innumerable, and I wouldn't trade those memories for anything.

According to Faceandbodydesign.com, driving has been shown to be very good for your mental state. Research has shown that getting behind the wheel of a car may reduce dementia risk and offer other health benefits for the elderly. As we age, we may also benefit from driving a car, both boosting cognitive function and staving off conditions like dementia. It may also halt the aging process. Had I only known, I could have stayed young forever.

Let's not forget that this country would be very different had it not been for the automobile. Driving a few miles on Route 66 or U.S. Highway 20 can give you an appreciation for the mass westward exodus from the East Coast city life America experienced. What would the 50s and 60s have been like without a car, drive-in theaters or drive-thru fast food restaurants like In-N-Out and A&W? I can tell you one thing, the West Coast would have been reserved only for the wealthy, as average families in the East and Midwest could only save up for annual western vacations.

No, driving is a guilty pleasure that I will hopefully never have to give up. With 85 being the new 65, I will do everything I can to be safely behind the wheel well beyond those years.

=================

I'll close with a quote from Tom Hanks: *"Growing up in northern California has had a big influence on my love and respect for the outdoors. When I lived in Oakland, we would think nothing of driving to Half Moon Bay and Santa Cruz one day and then driving to the foothills of the Sierras the next day."*

3. Museums

To some, a trip to a museum is an invitation to take a nap. How can a recreated bedroom from the 19th century possibly be interesting? Native American artifacts? Seen them. An actual Union Army uniform from the Civil War? Ho-hum.

Well, that's some people. Not us.

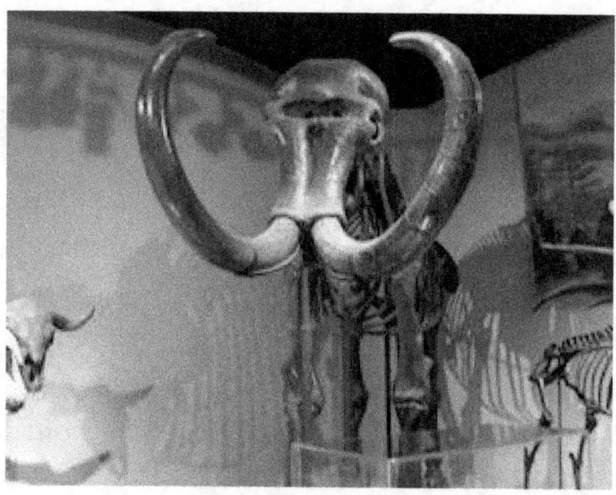

As we travel the country, one of the perks is to visit museums in different regions, often displaying items from the history of that specific area. My wife, Nadyne, is especially interested in historical museums and I very much enjoy art and natural history. In either case, we feel a special connection to nature and the past that we would not have enjoyed otherwise.

There is a peculiar feeling one can experience if they see or touch an item that is centuries old. One can imagine the people who may have made it, used it, painted it, wore it, lived in it or wrote about it, and realize they were not much different from us today. Enter a building marked, "Washington slept here," and one can feel the goose bumps thinking about occupying the same space now that the Father of our Country did in the 1700s. When I see a fossil or meteorite, I am in awe of the pure age of it.

When I was a kid, I vividly remember visiting two museums that filled me with awe and wonder. One was the Los Angeles Museum of Natural History, which was filled with fossils, both loose and those rebuilt into complete skeletons, complete collections of insects and rocks, and dioramas of people and settings all through the ages, from cavemen to present day. The other was the J. Paul Getty Museum, an extraordinary museum of classic and contemporary art. Both gave me feelings of belonging to the human race and connected me with the past that reading books could never duplicate.

Around the country, local museums proudly display artifacts found in the area or were donated by significant families with regional ties. Sometimes a visitor center can double as a museum, such as the Dry Falls Visitor Center in Washington State near the

Grand Coulee Dam. Displayed there are Native American artifacts and fossils from the Columbia River, and amazing exhibits and depictions of the massive ice age floods that shaped the region. In Wyoming and Colorado there are a variety of rural museums that highlight the struggles of the westward migration and the corresponding Native American ways of life.

In New England, you can't drive 10 minutes without seeing a museum focusing on the War of Independence or the Civil War. Up and down the East Coast, from Florida to Maine are maritime museums and scattered around the countryside are aviation and space museums. Across the South and East are those specializing in Black history, and they can be found in nearly every major city in America. Musicians and entertainers have whole industries based on preserving their past, and on-site filming locations for movies and television shows, often featuring their stars, have become popular destinations.

Last, no matter the sport you can find a historical center for it, and perhaps even a Hall of Fame. My preference is baseball, e.g., Cooperstown, N.Y., but I understand that you can also find my 808 three-game series in the U.S. Bowling Congress Hall of Fame.

All are fascinating, so, yes, museums make us happy. I don't think we'll ever get bored visiting them.

=================

I'll end this segment with an oft-heard and paraphrased quote by writer and philosopher George Santayana, who once said, "*Those who cannot remember the past are condemned to repeat it.*"

4. Pets

Not everyone loves pets. They can be a pain to feed, clean up after, train (if even possible), and keep safe and healthy. Did I mention the expense of feeding and keeping them healthy? Pets range from dogs and cats to birds, lizards, snakes, hamsters, fish and exotic beasts. Sizes can vary as well, with each pet family offering up a wide array of choices. Pet snakes might be a 2-foot garter snake or an 8-foot boa constrictor. A dog might be a chihuahua or a great Dane. Factor in lifestyle and the difficulties can expand exponentially.

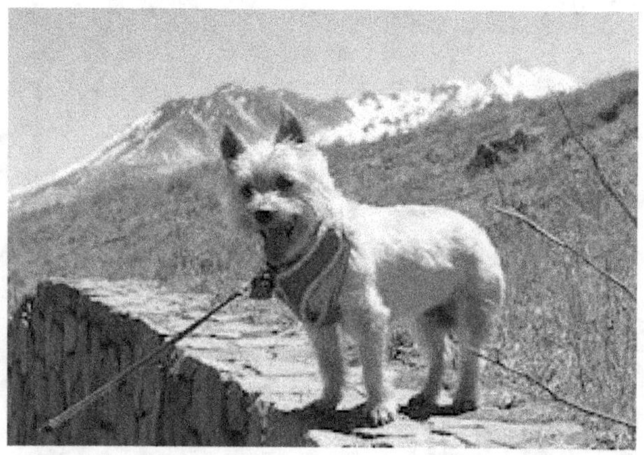

Losing a long-time pet companion, a member of the family, can be excruciating and can take years to recover, if at all. Unfortunately, like many pet owners, this has happened to me several times during my life. I remember the lyrics from Mr. Bojangles: "His dog up and died, he up and died, and after 20 years he still grieves." Most people we have talked to who have lost beloved pets fall into this category.

So, why have a pet? The simple answer is that they bring us joy. Though I'm partial to mammals and birds -- animals that have thinking brains -- I know of people with iguanas, turtles, frogs or even angelfish who believe that their pet companions love them.

Like many boys, I had a menagerie of animals as pets growing up. I even raised white lab rats. I've had a full spectrum of tropical fish, amphibians, reptiles, parakeets, rabbits, cats and dogs. I never liked snakes or live insects, and turtles were boring. I'm allergic to cats, so they have never been my choice, but in my mind they don't compare to dogs anyway. (Note to cat people: I'm not dissing cats. The tendencies and affections dogs show are just more my style.) I've never owned a horse, but my son and daughter-in-law have two.

Ask almost any dog owner what is the one thing is that their dogs do that makes them happy and they'll say the same thing — giving them unconditional love. If you doubt this, just say goodbye and leave the house, then return in two minutes to retrieve your keys and they will act like you've been gone all day. Come home from a terrible day at the office and they can show so much excitement to see you that your troubles can melt away.

There are science-backed benefits of owning a dog, and most apply to just about any pet. They make you feel less alone and can help you live longer. Studies suggest that dog owners have lower blood pressure levels and improved responses to stress. Active pets encourage or require you to move, something now considered mandatory for good health. An attractive pet, especially a dog, actually makes you more attractive to the opposite sex, with more phone numbers swapped and dates arranged when a pet is present than without one. Last, but not least, your pet can make you happier and more social.

We had the pleasure of visiting my daughter and her partner in Seattle last summer and I was a little worried before arriving. I knew they had parakeets and a cockatiel that they let fly free in their house. I needn't have been concerned. They loved us.

==================

As a cute finishing thought, I'll turn to Novelist Anne Tyler. *"Ever consider what pets must think of us? I mean, here we come back from a grocery store with the most amazing haul - chicken, pork, half a cow. They must think we're the greatest hunters on earth!"*

5. Acts of Kindness

The topic of kindness might be particularly timely given the current political climate. We, myself included, need to remember that we are human beings first, then all else. All humans depend upon other humans for their survival and quality of life. I know it can be difficult, but that's part of the purpose of these discussions.

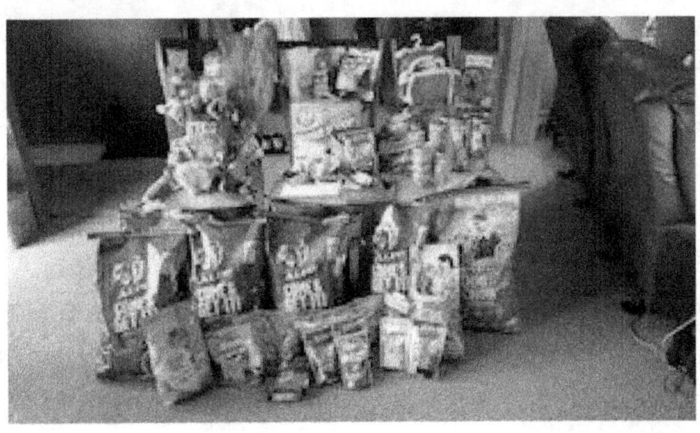

I have always tried to do the little things to show kindness, like opening doors for people (man, woman or child), donating time to charities or a worthy organization, returning found money, giving rides and many others. I once took a temporary job for half my normal pay because it was for a non-profit business helping the blind. Throughout my career, I have volunteered for a variety of projects and tasks that were helping people who were homeless or lower income. I have had my fast food order paid by the car in front of me and have paid for the order of the car in line behind me. I believe in the concept of paying it forward.

We have also received kindness. A few years ago, after we bought our fifth wheel but before we went full time, we hosted an outing for our camping club in Eagle's Nest, New Mexico. We were among the last to depart at the end of the long weekend, and just has we hit Trinidad, Colorado, over five hours from home, the radiator burst on my pickup. We scrambled to find somewhere to repair it, but since it was Sunday, this took time. We finally found a repair shop that would look at it the next day, but we had to be at work that Monday and had to find a way to get home. We texted friend after friend to see if they were nearby, but all our camping buddies had passed Trinidad a bit earlier. One couple, though, told us to stay put and wait. They were 85 miles north of us, but unhooked their rig and drove the hour-and-a-half to pick us up. We stopped back at their fifth wheel to re-hook-up and drive the last three hours home. To top off this incredibly selfless act, they loaned us their car for as long as it would take to retrieve the truck.

There are many ways you can begin to perform little acts of kindness. Give a compliment to someone, especially someone struggling, or point out a positive for them. Tell them that they matter. Volunteer or contribute to a charity. I find there is more satisfaction in helping than just writing a check. Listen to someone actively respond to what they are saying. Put yourself in their place. They may need that, and this shows that you understand what they are going through, which can help make them feel better. Help someone who didn't think to ask you. Solve a problem for someone or teach them a new skill. Start a new project or initiative toward social good. Analyze if a product or company is ethical and react accordingly. Stand for something. Say "thank you."

The Good Samaritan couple that helped us in Trinidad is a perfect example of the few who regularly perform acts of kindness. Their actions continuously motivate others to do the same. Together we can all help make the world a better place, and that, people, should make you happy.

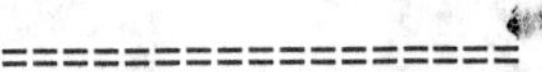

As a closing thought, I'll quote Ellen DeGeneres: *"Here are the values that I stand for: honesty, equality, kindness, compassion, treating people the way you want to be treated and helping those in need. To me, those are traditional values."*

6. The Celestial Sky

From the time I first starting reading, I was looking through astronomy textbooks. I remember seeing a photograph of Mars and its maze of straight lines, thought to be canals. We now know, of course, that it was a false image. But it fascinated me. When I was a pre-teen, I made my own telescope out of a cardboard tube, tape and a couple of lenses I saved my allowance to buy. It actually worked OK, until it fell apart. Once in high school, I visited the planetarium at Griffith Park in Los Angeles as often as I could.

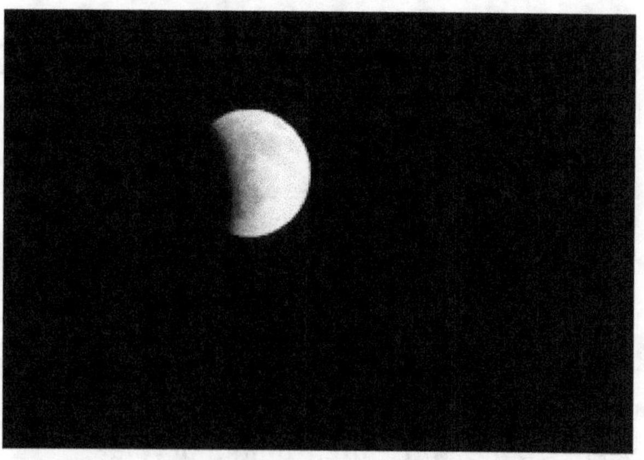

After I became a family man and moved to Washington State, I bought my own telescope, expensive at the time, and was amazed at the actual sight of Jupiter with four of its moons and Saturn and its rings, though they were in a flat plane at the time. My problem was that without an expensive actuator to move the device along with the sky's movement, objects only stayed in my field of view for a few moments. A few years later, living in Colorado, I always enjoyed visiting our friends in rural Wyoming, where on clear summer nights far removed from any city light, the Milky Way was so brilliant that we couldn't make out the constellations.

This past year in Colorado, we were camped in a remote RV resort about 75 miles from the nearest city lights and the Milky Way again was visible. There was an amateur astronomer camping in the park and one night he set up his equipment for any of us to view. We saw Jupiter, this time with five moons visible, Uranus' striped globe, Saturn's awesome rings tilted down at 45 degrees, and some nebulae and spiral galaxies. It was an amazing night that nearly brought me to tears.

"Celestial sky" can be defined as the sky between dusk and dawn during the time stars and other celestial objects can be seen. Sunshine, obviously, makes it impossible to see stars and planets, but you'd be surprised to see how much difference being away from the city can make, and even having a new moon or no moon can make the sky astounding. There are several exciting phone apps you can now use to decipher the stars and planets above you, even those in the sky during the day, when they are invisible. I use StarTracker, but there are others.

In my life I have seen the Aurora Boealis, several lunar eclipses and a blood moon, a nearly full solar eclipse, two comets, and a meteorite that lit up the night sky like daylight — I have even taken my kids to watch the Perseid Meteor Shower — all with awe. The bottom line is that when I contemplate what I am seeing when I view Jupiter, the Milky Way or even the moon, I feel an emotional tug of pleasure, sometimes overwhelming, and am awestruck. The sheer distance and age, the wonder, the possibility of other intelligent life out there that humans will probably never discover, the beginning and the end of the universe -- I see it all and think, wow!

==================

I'll close this topic with a quote from British scientist Martin Rees, who wrote, "*Indeed, the night sky is the part of our environment that's been common to all cultures throughout human history. All have gazed up at the 'vault of heaven' and interpreted it in their own way.*"

7. Wild Birds

They provide the city with nature and music to an otherwise quiet forest, sometimes with a cacophony. As wildlife goes, birds are relatively benign, unlike moose, bears or snakes, and there is such a variety that endless communities of birdwatchers never tire of searching for and pondering them. Even as a boy and newly-supplied with my first black-and-white camera, I loved photographing birds.

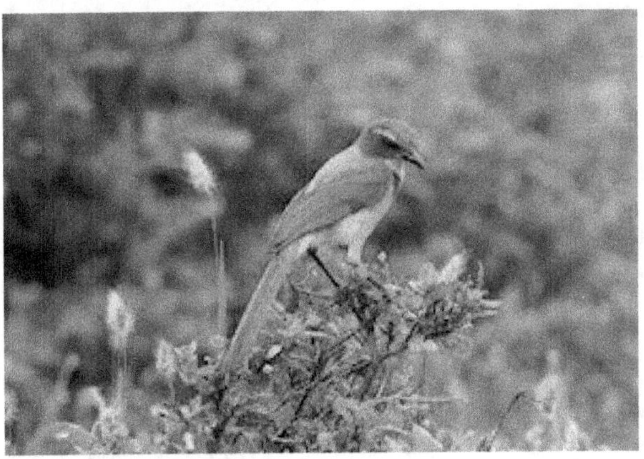

I remember the first time I saw an eagle in the wild, a massive golden eagle in the Mojave Desert that seemed to stand about as tall as my 12-year-old body at the time. It was about a quarter mile away, and we stopped and watched as it was joined by another gargantuan specimen with an unfortunate victim clutched in a claw. Obviously a mated pair, they wrestled for a few minutes on the ground before majestically taking to the cloudless blue sky. I had been hiking with other Boy Scouts and didn't have my camera, but I knew there would be a lifetime of opportunities in my life. I was right.

I often think about mammals having thinking brains, unlike most other types of life on the planet, but the more you watch wild birds the more you realize that they must also be thinking. They watch their surroundings, contemplate their options, then decide whether to flee, fight or try something new. I've seen jay birds figure out, after several attempts, how to open a squirrel feeder, and robins team up to fight off some annoying grackles. They amaze me.

There have been many sightings of intelligence in birds. In Japan, carrion crows will place nuts on roadways for cars to run over. Woodpecker finches have been seen trimming twigs to the proper length to use in foraging for insects. Herons have been known to use bread and other scraps to attract fish for hunting. They can often recognize who is filling bird feeders, and interact with different people differently. Watching birds and witnessing their intelligent behavior can be a joy for birders.

Speaking of birding, I have been using the Cornell University site, ebird.com, to post photos and checklists of bird species found in various outings. However, it might take me 10 different sites to locate the species of a specific bird I've photographed, and sometimes even then I'm unable to determine it with some accuracy and confidence. It is fun, though, and I'll continue to share my findings.

Many times, I have seen a bird of an uncommon species, like a yellow-headed blackbird or painted bunting, only to have it fly away as I scramble for my camera, even if it was close by. Perhaps it was the only time in my life to see a member of that species live and up close, and I have to be satisfied with the single viewing.

==================

I'll close these musings with a quote from British journalist David Attenborough: "*Everyone likes birds. What wild creature is more accessible to our eyes and ears, as close to us and everyone in the world, as universal as a bird?*"

8. Movie Theaters

My first ever experience in a movie theater occurred when I was about 10 years old. One of my friends had a birthday party on a sunny Saturday afternoon at an indoor theater playing *Help!* with the Beatles. A few years later, my best friend's parents took us to see Clint Eastwood's *Play Misty For Me* in a drive-in, the first time I had seen a movie in that venue. Both impacted me greatly, and I have cherished those memories for years. Before that time, television was the only media I had witnessed. Compared to the theater, TV was drivel.

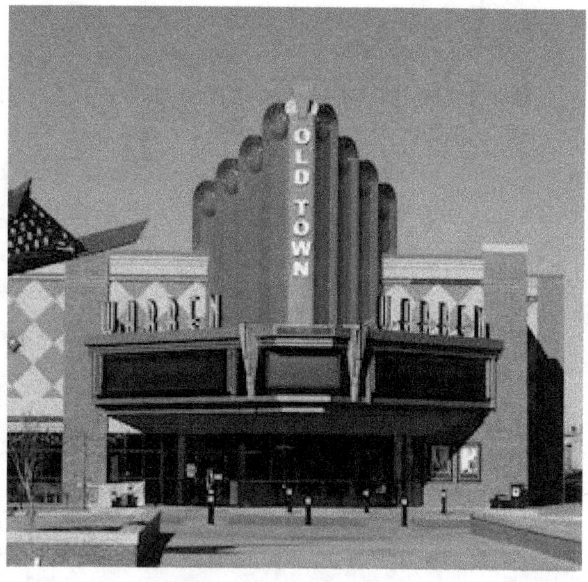

As a teenager I saw many B movies in the local indoor joint, the Star Theater, and we would waste the whole day seeing both movies (they used to show double-features) twice, all for one ticket price, which I think was three bucks. Horror and science fiction flicks could be seen in the 60s for a mere 50 cents all day on Sundays. I saw *Them!*, *The Day the Earth Stood Still*, Bela Legosi's *Dracula*, various renditions of Frankenstein's monster, Steve McQueen's *The Blob*, several episodes of *Dark Shadows*, and many other classics in that old theater made out of a World War II barracks .

A couple of premiers stand out in my mind. I saw the original *Star Wars* flick in a drive-in on its 1977 opening day, and I waited in line for three hours to see *Independence Day* (the Will Smith alien movie) on its July 4, 1996, opening day. That was long-awaited, since they began promoting it the Thanksgiving before.

There is something special about sharing a movie experience with a larger group of people. Kids at theaters weren't breaking windows or vandalizing cars, and many life lessons could be learned at the movies. The popcorn was always hot and buttery, though expensive, and the big screen was just that — BIG. The best part, though, was the simultaneous reactions of a crowd watching a movie together. I remember sharing non-stop laughs in *What's Up Doc?* and *Airplane!*, which was the first movie where I ever saw my dad laugh, and standing with the entire audience in a unified gasp during

Harold and Maude when Harold's awesome Jaguar/Hearse drove off a cliff. The buildup and fear of *The Exorcist* would have been so much less if it weren't shared and anticipated by a full theater of horror fans.

A series of well-made war movies, starting with *The Deer Hunter, Apocalypse Now, Patton, Good Morning, Viet Nam*, and eventually *Schindler's List*, placed reality and plot above heroism and gave people new insights into the war machine. To this day I can still hear the loud whine of the phone melting in Henry Fonda's *Fail Safe*, as the American diplomat in Moscow and his office was hit by a nuclear blast.

My favorite movies include *Contact, Paint Your Wagon, Kelly's Heroes, The Natural, The Day of the Jackal* and *Grand Canyon*. If I made a complete list of movies I loved, however, it would probably consist of 300 or more.

Large screen TV's and sound systems make it more convenient to watch a movie in full surround sound that shakes the living room, and while there is something to be said for the pause button when you have to run to the bathroom, what is lost, like the massive 70-foot coated projection screen and a full room of those sharing the experience, is so meaningful.

==================

I'll finish off my blog post with a quote from film maker Steven Spielberg: "*I love to go to a regular movie theater, especially when the movie is a big crowd-pleaser. It's much better watching a movie with 500 people making noise than with just a dozen.*"

9. Sense of Smell

I don't think our sense of smell gets enough kudos. Sure, the sweet scent of a flower or a fabulous meal can enhance an experience, and the stink of a big fish can be the result of a successful outing or vacation. Terrible smells, such as skunk or rotten eggs, serve their purpose as well, helping identify potential danger or alarming situations. But there's more going on.

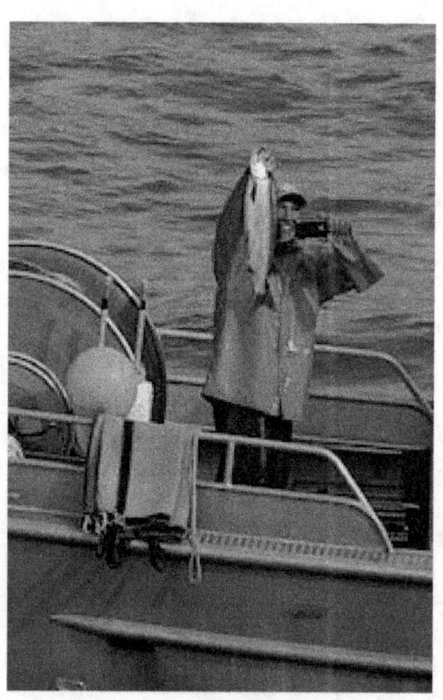

It turns out that the parts of the brain that handle smell, emotion and memories are closely intertwined. This makes smell the most directly connected of our five senses to specific memories.

With emotions attached, very often happy or pleasing events are quickly conjured up with a particular scent. They added a scent to natural gas for this very purpose.

Our ability to smell is due to airborne molecules activating olfactory receptors in the nasal cavities. These molecules must be vaporized and also have some solubility in water. Receptors convert the molecules into various patterns, which are sent to the brain. The pattern of signals arriving at the brain constitutes the 'smell' of the molecule perceived by the brain. Since an animal's survival may depend upon these smells, bad smells are generally universal. What constitutes a good smell, however, may depend on the person's association in a positive sense, even if it is a scent of a skunk. Humans have about 5 to 6 million olfactory receptors, compared with 220 million in dogs and 100 million in rabbits, but I have yet to see a smell-tracking rabbit. That would be cool, though.

My own experiences bear this out. When I smell a vinyl record, I am immediately transported to 1969 and listening to a brand new 45 (a vinyl record with a song on each side, played on a device called a record player) I had just purchased with my allowance, *And When I Die* by Blood, Sweat and Tears. I was sleeping over at my friend's house, his driveway, really, as we were staying in his dad's pickup camper. We played that song until the smell of roasting marshmallows from the back yard gained our attention.

The smell of processed film, the media we used in cameras before digital photography always takes me back to my grandmother's house when I was 10 years old. She had just given me her Brownie camera, my first, and helped me load the film. Similarly, the smell of burning wood brings memories of the first time I took my kids tent camping over a long weekend up in Washington State. Happy memories indeed.

The smells of love are probably the most pleasing, with the scents of sweat, perfume, wine, or shared food bringing happy memories immediately to mind. Similarly, there are a number of scents that can benefit your well-being. Lavender is said to help someone sleep, cinnamon can sharpen your mind, and pine can alleviate stress. Fresh cut grass can make you more joyful, though it makes me sneeze. Citrus can energize you, vanilla can raise your mood and pumpkin, believe it or not, can be an aphrodisiac.

There is a lot to be happy about when considering the sense of smell, one of the senses that can warn you of danger before it is in sight, and bring back your most precious memories with one small whiff.

==================

I'll end this essay with a quote from the consummate American author, Helen Keller: *"Smell is a potent wizard that transports you across thousands of miles and all the years you have lived."*

10. Craft Beer

They used to call me a wine snob, but I didn't think of myself that way. There weren't many wines I wouldn't drink, only the sweetest whites or dessert wines. I had spent considerable time in wine country, both in Washington State and New York State, and I picked up a few things, right? I never liked beer and it even took a while for me to acquire a taste for wine.

Back in my karaoke days, I became aware of how blood alcohol content testing can affect someone's life. I was naturally reticent to drink more than two glasses of wine in an evening before driving home, and shots of any hard alcohol were out of the question. But I was still thirsty and was forced to drink water to finish out the night. Water was not great for vocal chords, at least not mine, and wasn't exactly tasty.

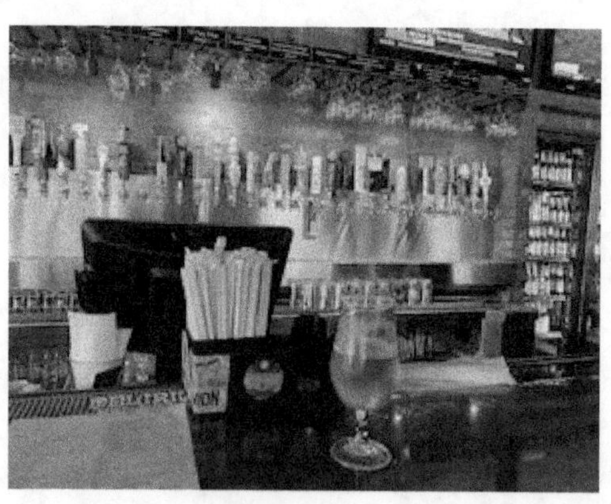

I began playing in traveling pool leagues where the beer was always flowing in whatever bar we were playing. Wine, not so much. I still had the issue of driving after drinking wine anyway, so I made the decision to try to attain a taste of beer, at least enough to drink with friends. I planned my assault on the project, deciding to start with apple ales, then graduate to light beer with lime before tasting a wider variety. The first couple of apple ales tasted good but were far too sweet and I quickly jumped to light beer, first with lime, then without. After a few weeks of Bud Light, I was unsure how to widen my horizon. Enter craft breweries.

I don't remember which microbrewery I tried but I tasted a few brews with mixed success. One weekend I was camping with our RV group in Colorado and my brother had joined us. Paul has always enjoyed beer and was happy to join me in a local brewery for samples. I obviously knew about flights of wines but had been unaware that beers could be ordered that way as well, at least at larger brewpubs and at breweries themselves. I tasted my first flight and began my beer adventures, determining what kind of beers I enjoy and which I dislike.

Just like with wine, where a novice may begin with a sweeter white wine like a Riesling and over time their tastes change, I found this to be the case with beer as well. I immediately disliked IPAs with their hoppy taste and any ales with citrus taste, especially sour.

Congregating to drink beer can be beneficial to one's life, according to Time Magazine. "A recent study ... found that having a regular watering hole helps improve social skills, which increases overall life satisfaction. According to the study, people who patronized a local or community-type pub or bar had a wider support system of close friends, which also meant that they were more trusting of others and more engaged with the community than those who did not support a local bar."

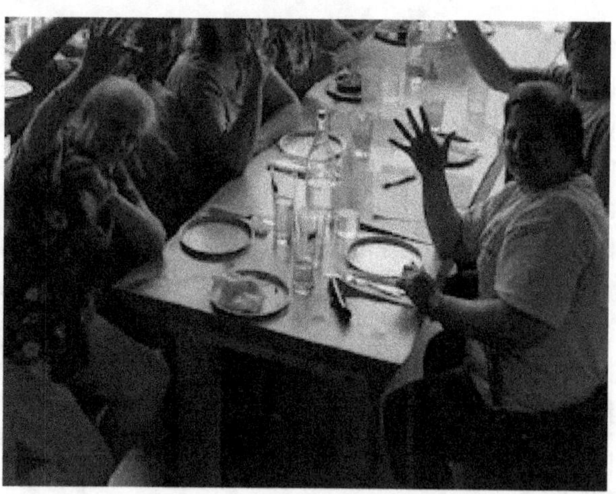

Here's a quick rundown on the various beer styles: Pale Lager and Pilsner, Dark Lager, German Bock, Brown Ale, Pale Ale, India Pale Ale, Belgian-Style Ale, Wheat Beer, Porter, Stout, Wild & Sour Ale and Specialty Beer. Within each are sub-categories, and unconventional or playful brewmeisters may mix styles or add their own unique signature and make a beer their own. Thus, even experienced beer connoisseurs can find new and exciting brews in any of the 8,000+ micro-breweries in the U.S. Even the big boys have joined the party, with major labels gobbling up many of the most popular craft breweries for their own lines.

I know many people who enjoy going into a large-volume liquor store or specialty beer outlet and spend afternoons mixing and matching cans, bottles, crawlers or growlers of the various makers of their favorite styles. There are brewery snobs who will only purchase beer from a single micro-brewery. I myself like to mix it up and will buy six-packs of different craft beers to take home. But, for me, draft beer ("draught" for the purists) is so superior to canned or bottled beer that I make sports bars or breweries a destination whenever I can. I am especially disappointed when I go out for dinner and the restaurant doesn't have draft, or the only drafts they have are light beers. Sadly, the pandemic made having draft beers next to impossible.

After a few years of sampling and drinking beer, I find myself drawn to Dark Lagers, red and brown Ales, Belgium-style Ales, Bocks, dry Irish Stouts and, in a pinch, Blond Ales. The one problem with traveling the country and visiting micro-breweries is that I will sometimes find a beer I love and can't buy anywhere else. That happened the last time we were in Maine, where I was drawn by a street full of bright red umbrellas at every restaurant, all with the same brewery's name, and found myself at their walk-up bar. Their dark lager was the best I've ever had, even to this day, and haven't found it anywhere outside of Maine. I'm looking forward to our return!

So, long story short, I had an aversion beer, I taught myself to drink the beverage and now I love certain styles of beer, especially when made by craft breweries. Like wine, there are so many varieties that one may never get bored having to stick to a certain style. In this way, beer can do many things to make someone happy. And, I only consumed 17.3 oz. of the stuff while writing this...

==================

I'll leave this discussion with a very astute quote from American author W. Bruce Cameron, who wrote, "*I've read that the ancient Chinese art of feng shui can bring a sense of peace, well-being, and positive energy to a home - same as beer.*"

11. Wildflowers

Our lifestyle, as we continue to tour the country, has provided an abundance of opportunities to enjoy wildflowers every day. I would venture to say I have more photos saved of wildflowers than any other single subject, and the colors draw from a palette of millions. There are a couple of themes that stick with me as we come across them.

One sentiment I often feel is that at least some of these floral organisms will grow in any environment we run across, from arid desert heat to ice-covered rock face, dark forest bed, wet marshland, rainforest, sandy beach or dry riverbed. Nature seems to adapt to any situation. In high-elevation settings you'll see miniature alpine blossoms. On a rocky cliff side, you'll often see multi-colored lichen overtaken by moss, then vines with soft pastel flowers. Even most desert cacti bloom annually.

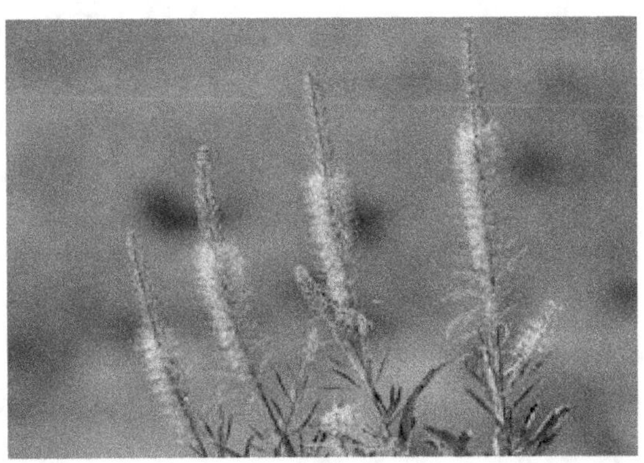

Another is the sheer variety of color, size, shape and brilliance of wildflowers, depending on what is needed for them to be successful where they are. Most require pollination by bees, moths, butterflies, hummingbirds or other nectar feeders, and it's not difficult to see that the variety aids in their survival and helps spread their species. Even the wind can determine the type of wildflowers you will find, with those stems and flowers that can bend and resist destruction being more prevalent in gusty regions.

Interestingly, some flowers can be found across the U.S., while others are specific to one locale. It can be comforting to see wild sunflowers, coneflowers or musk mallows everywhere you drive, a sort of continuity that can sooth the awkward exploration of a new location. On the other hand, it can be exciting to see Texas bluebonnets, California poppies, Colorado columbines or the yellow jessamines of the Carolinas.

Once all flowers were wildflowers. They have been beautifying the earth for over 130 million years, sustaining a complex mixture of interdependent systems, insects and other wildlife. During winter months, when there is less food available for wildlife, wildflower seeds can be an important food source for birds and small mammals.

They provide soil erosion protection, seemingly oblivious to all sorts of extreme weather. Some are native to the land in which they live, while many were brought by people in other parts of the world. All non-native plants are considered invasive, so we must make sure we do not move any plants into a region in which they are not native. Wildflowers also contribute to scientific and medical research and some wildflowers contain compounds that can be used in drugs to treat diseases. For example, foxgloves contain chemicals used to treat cardiac issues.

You may ask what the difference is between weeds and wildflowers. Weeds are plants that are in the wrong place and often compete for resources with nearby plants. Wildflowers are in their natural setting and aren't usually competitive enough to be considered problematic.

==================

I'll finish up the topic by sharing a quote from a famous American author, John Steinbeck: "*Men do change, and change comes like a little wind that ruffles the curtains at dawn, and it comes like the stealthy perfume of wildflowers hidden in the grass.*"

12. Sunrise

There are some obvious, even cliché, feelings everyone has about sunrise, at least in some point in their lives. It symbolizes a brand-new start, of leaving yesterday behind and the promise of good things to come. I have those feelings, too, but wanted to delve deeper. There's something else about watching a sunrise, something visceral.

First, compared to sunsets, the colors and radiance of sunrises are often more brilliant at sunrise. This may be because of atmospheric conditions in which haze and smog can build all day, leaving sunsets muted, albeit sometimes with a wider palette. Also, the sun approaching the horizon has its rays slowly building until the first light leaps in a blinding shine of light. With the opposite trajectory, the sunlight fades from its last direct light of the day. These might be comparable to your eyes, depending on conditions, but emotionally the former is more exciting.

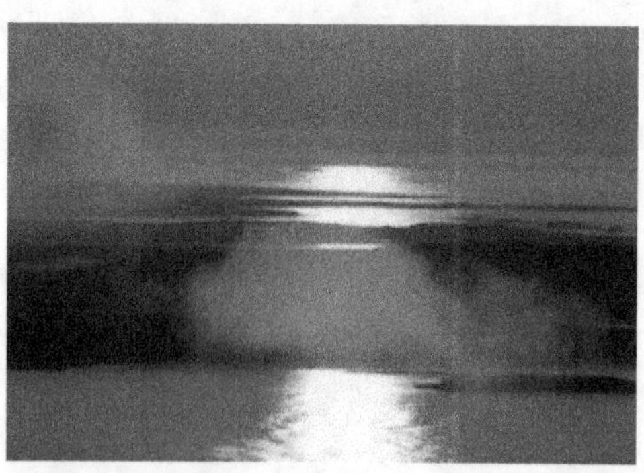

Comparisons would not be fair without considering the landscape at the location you choose. The shape, type and abundance of clouds can make or break either daybreak or day's end, so very often you do have to be in the right place at the right time. Too many, too thick or too few clouds can ruin the photogenic aspects of the shot. In Florida, you have the best opportunity for great sunrises on the Atlantic shore and for wonderful sunsets on the Gulf shore. In Colorado, sunrises east of the Rockies will be much better than sunsets due to the extremely high horizon -- the sun never gives the vivid hues because it has already set behind the mountains. I've always loved both sunrise and sunset over large bodies of water, so my best photos depend on that -- sunrise in Maine, sunset at the eastern shore of Lake Ontario in Upstate New York. All of that said, coastal regions suffer fog or marine layers that often eliminate sunrises completely. That was true often during our travel through New England.

For some, sunrise can be a religious experience, or at least a confirmation of the awesome God they pray to. I'm not religious, but I felt the sunrise I witnessed from Cadillac Mountain in Acadia National Park definitely had a spiritual aura, something I shared with about 2,000 other tourists and photographers.

There are numerous positive effects from watching a sunrise. You will probably be in a better mood throughout the day after the experience, and it has been proven to help fight stress, depression and anxiety. It might also make you grateful for the earth and nature. Though it is a daily experience, every sunrise is different, with a myriad of environmental aspects affecting the sight. Not only do you have all of those aspects, you get them all for free.

Take all the science, the fact that I am up early to watch, the emotional clichés and crisp, brilliant colors, and I'd have to say that sunrise is always something special and my preference. Yes, I have taken some amazing sunset photos, but just as many sunrises have made my favorites list and the other factors I've mentioned make the difference.

==================

I'll end this discussion with a quote from a 19th century leader in New Zealand, George Grey: *"Sunrise offered a very beautiful spectacle; the water was quite unruffled, but the motion communicated by the tides was so great that, although there was not a breath of air stirring, the sea heaved slowly with a grand and majestic motion."*

13. Enjoying Retirement

For most, retirement is a phase of life, a chapter near the end of the book, a distinct change in lifestyle. Social Security age requirements may influence the target (retire at 62, wait until full benefits kick in or decide on something in between), or perhaps the status of one's 401K or retirement savings plan, or more importantly, one's health condition. Any way you get there, hopefully you can enjoy it.

My father passed away from a stroke at age 55, and he had huge retirement plans that he never had a chance to fulfill. My wife's mother became ill just about when her father retired, and he put aside their retirement travel plans. When he tragically passed away before her, she was still too weak to travel. That inspired both of us to retire and hit the road running as soon as possible. I did postpone my exit as a manager a few months until I could help train my replacement, but was still 62 and Nadyne 63 when we pulled the trigger, selling our house and moving into our fifth wheel.

We had planned our escape for five years and could hardly believe when it finally arrived. Downsizing was far more difficult than we expected, and leaving friends behind was equally disheartening.

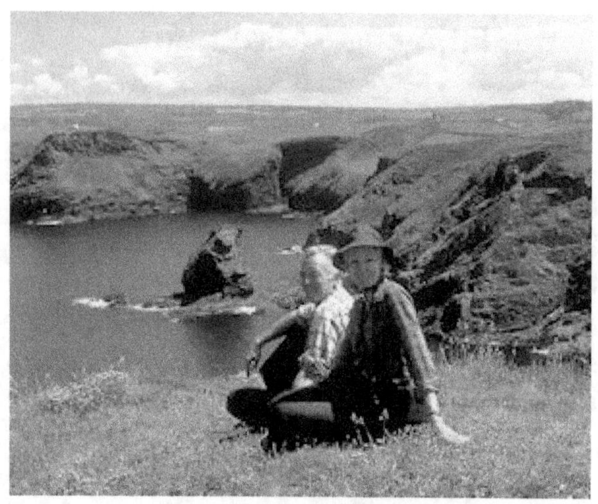

Social Security only pays so much and we have resisted using savings, so Nadyne is still working about 40 hours per month and I am writing books and articles so that we can be more comfortable in our travel.

Since retiring and moving to the highways and byways of America, we have had good times and bad, the latter mostly having to do with our RV repairs, losing Lucy, our beloved dog of 12 years, and COVID restrictions. However, the sights we've seen, the experiences we've shared, the awe of nature, the splendor of the night sky, and the interesting differences in landscape and community among the different sections of the country — all of these have made our lifestyle much more than satisfying. As an added bonus, we've been able to visit, in person, our six kids, five grandchildren, four great-grandchildren, and 10 siblings and their families, scattered across the country. This would not have been possible if we weren't able to retire and travel freely like we do.

I did not experience a culture shock when I stopped getting up at 4:45 a.m. on weekdays. Instead, I began to "sleep in" until 7 a.m. and stay up as long as I like. Sometimes I even stay in bed until 8:30! Before the pandemic, we were able to experience the local night life and regional restaurant favorites wherever we happened to be and I have now sung karaoke in about 20 states. I now have photo galleries posted from 35 states and our two cruises (Alaska and the Caribbean), much of which has been taken since we hit the road. We return to Colorado every summer to catch up with friends and do the doctor and dentist routines, as well as touring one of our favorite states.

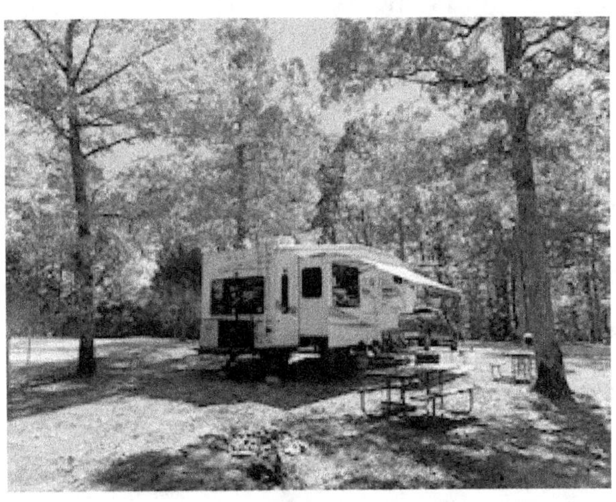

And then there are the myriad of friendships we've made, some due to our membership and activities in RVillage (now approaching 400,000 RV members), and some are people we meet along our journeys. The RV community is an unusual bunch in that members have much more in common than not. Almost everyone has stories about a black tank experience or a particularly bizarre campground, and they can't wait to share experiences with people who haven't heard them yet and want to share their own stories. We see a few of our RV friends in multiple locations, which is always fun. One couple has crossed our path in Pennsylvania, Florida, Texas and Ohio, and another in California, Florida and Oregon.

None of this would have been possible without our retiring while we still had our health. Sadly, like both of our fathers, some never get the chance. I highly recommend it!

==================

Most quotes I find about retirement are either political or financial in nature. However, British actor Richard C. Armitage had this to say: "*My instruction to my parents is that I would rather they enjoy their retirement than leave me anything when they go. I am much happier watching them enjoying life.*" Mr. Armitage, I salute you.

14. Rain

As long as I can remember, I've loved the rain. Contrary to popular belief, it does rain in Southern California, but as a kid it was even better when it poured. I could hardly wait until I could go outside and get soaking wet. Springtime brought the rain back then, and the old adage seemed to be true: April showers bring May flowers.

There are many more reasons I love the rain now. Having lived through severe droughts, rain still brings an almost automatic reflex of relief. It is the one weather event that happens worldwide, so it can help you feel connected to the earth no matter where you are, much like seeing the moon or stars can do for you at night. It represents sustaining life in so many ways.

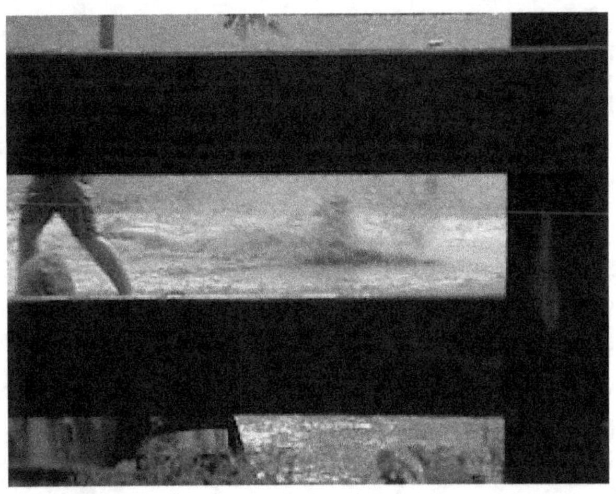

Living beings require water to live, even more than food, and rain is how we get all of our fresh water. A shower can give a sense of cleansing, of washing away the grime of life, of washing away our sins. After a good rain, our mood is almost always lifted. There is a reason for the popularity of *Dancing in the Rain*. During a drenching rain storm, most of us are forced to stay indoors, giving us an excuse to snuggle up with our mate or kids in front of a fire, drink hot chocolate, make some popcorn and watch a new or a favorite movie. Stormy nights remind us of the power and awe of nature, of the good and bad of it, and this is exaggerated when roaring thunder shakes the house.

Rain pours through the atmosphere, cooling and humidifying hot air, warming ambient cold air in winter months, and clings to specks of pollution to literally condition the air around us. It moisturizes your skin and cleanses plant leaves. It adds moisture to farms' soil, helps leach salts down beyond the root zone and the rivers it creates are dammed for hydroelectric power.

But the thing I like most about the rain is its sound. If you've never fallen to sleep to the soothing pitter-patter of rain on the roof above you, you've really missed out. Of course, a hard rain or hail pounding on a metal roof can be deafening but awe-inspiring.

Ever notice how quickly the scenery greens up after a summer rain? Is there anything more precious than seeing a group of school-aged children in rain coats and boots stomping in puddles? Every see a child's face the first time you tell them that it's raining cats and dogs? Interestingly, the source of that phrase is unknown. It might have its roots in Norse mythology, medieval superstitions, the obsolete word catadupe (waterfall), or dead animals in the streets of Britain being picked up by storm waters. We do know that Richard Brome, an English playwright, wrote in his 1652 comedy, *City Witt*, "It shall rain dogs and polecats." However, a polecat back then was more related to a weasel than a cat.

What I miss most about living in Kansas are the summer storms. Though often severe, we haven't experienced anything even close to it since we moved away. It always reminded me that without rain, there is no rainbow.

==================

My closing quote for this topic is from American poet Langston Hughes, who wrote, "*Let the rain kiss you. Let the rain beat upon your head with silver liquid drops. Let the rain sing you a lullaby.*"

15. Best Friends

One of the common threads between people of all walks of life is that of having one or more best friends. It is quite possible to maintain this type of connection throughout one's life, even as other types of relationships come and go. Most of the outstanding marriages I have seen are between best friends.

With most people, their first bestie comes along very young, possibly in kindergarten or first grade. Life is difficult, as are older siblings, if any, and sharing good and bad times with a friend is as natural as breathing. I'm no psychologist, but I imagine that the tendency to seek out a best friend is hardwired into our collective psyche. Life happens, and sometimes very young friends are separated by moving, a falling out or simply growing apart. This happens with grade school friends, too, even with high school friends, but the older they get, the more best friends are apt to stay in contact. College or adult life, work, recreation and other natural gathering places may supply multiple very good friends and the ones that stick it out through bad times often become your favorites.

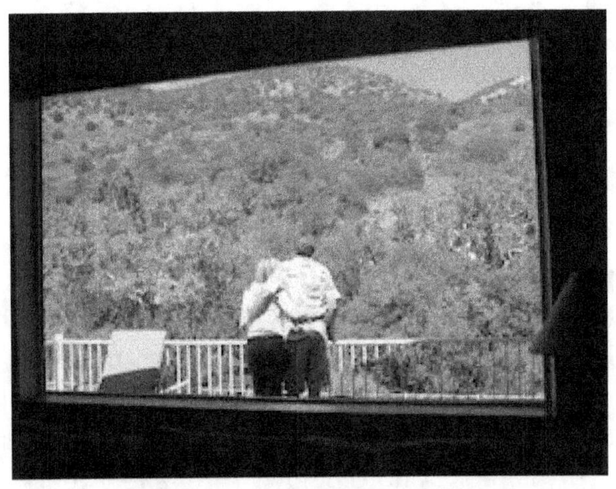

The one prerequisite "best friends" seem to have is to support one another despite the circumstances -- always having each other's back. You don't owe one another any favors. In fact, you don't even keep count. Fair weather friends just can't compete for your time and attention. When a best friend calls, you drop everything. Maybe this is why best friends make such good married or committed couples.

My first best friend was Kenny Hakida when I was 5 years old. He lived next door to my grandparents, which was a long, two-mile walk from my house at the time. We moved 40 miles away when I was 10 and I never saw Kenny again. I later learned that his parents had been among those Japanese-Americans interned in World War II after

Pearl Harbor, but I never got the chance to talk to them about it.

I had a few other best friends in my adolescence and in high school in Southern California, but many of them went to out-of-state colleges, while I got married and had kids. Moving a thousand miles away meant the end of most of those relationships. In Washington State, my younger brother filled that role, through bowling, karaoke, camping, fishing and other activities we both enjoyed. He's the taller one in my karaoke photo below. After a few years I moved across the country to be close to, and eventually marry, my present and last best friend.

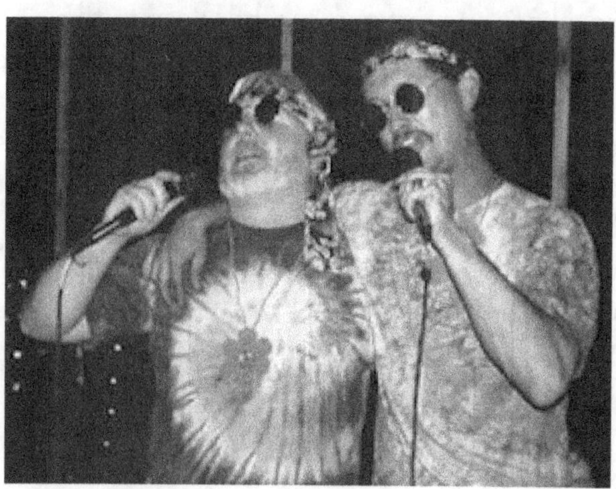

I envy the good friends of today, with all of that technology available to help stay in touch. In my younger days, even long-distance phone calls were very expensive, let alone trying to see one another.

If we had had the Internet, free long distance, Facebook, Zoom, Skype, GroupMe or any other of the seemingly magical communications they have now, maybe my old friends wouldn't be strangers today.

Thankfully, my wife and I had each other to lean on in close quarters during the pandemic lockdown. If it weren't for that relationship, who knows how well we would have survived it.

=================

My ending quote comes from an Israeli psychologist, Daniel Kahneman, who said, "*Friends are sometimes a big help when they share your feelings. In the context of decisions, the friends who will serve you best are those who understand your feelings but are not overly impressed by them.*"

16. Country Fairs

According to Wikipedia, the first known agricultural show was held by Salford Agricultural Society, Lancashire, in 1768. Lancashire is a county in a far northern section of England. Agricultural shows evolved to country fairs and, in America, they are mostly state and county fairs. These annual events usually include a livestock show and auction, a trade fair, competitions among local residents, and entertainment, including live music by local artists and headliners, a carnival and a great many vendors serving what is now called "fair food." Often a rodeo is held in conjunction with the fair, and we've even seen auto racing, monster truck shows and demolition derbies get in on the event calendars. Let's not forget about the carnival rides and midway.

We usually avoid state fairs because they are usually more crowded than their county cousins. It is especially fun to visit rural, small-town fairs. The entertainment is not normally nationally headlining acts, but I have seen Roger Miller, the Smothers and Righteous Brothers (an awesome combination), Little River Band, Anne Murray and other previously big-time artists in the smaller venues.

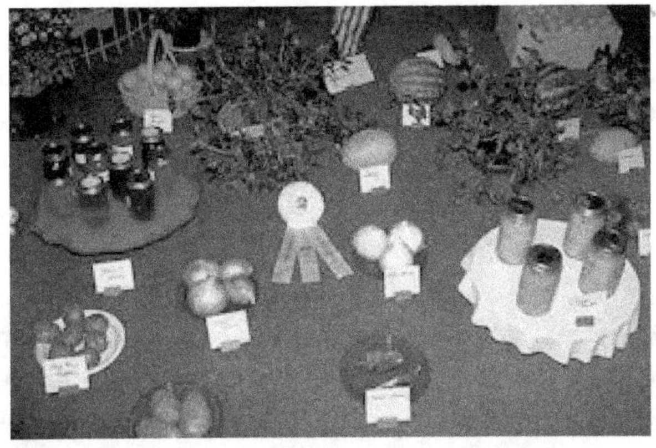

Otherwise, my favorite sections in the fair are the animals being shown and the collections of all kinds, including the most random things you can think of. Besides the usual (e.g., rocks, gems, quilts, stamps and coins), we've seen *Wizard of Oz* and *Gone With the Wind* memorabilia, antique camping gear, and even dryer lint collections. You just never know what you're going to see. Local residents yearning to win a blue ribbon is not just a cliché. Many spend hours and hours all year to compete in their chosen hobby, be it baking, sewing, pickling, floral arrangement or other skill, and the quality of their displays and products is usually quite remarkable.

Fair food has become its own genre, and many fairs compete with the craziest things they could batter and deep fry. The last one we attended had just begun to serve deep-fried beer and deep-fried butter. Often, though, fair favorites are fresh corn-on-the-cob, funnel cakes, corn dogs and the always popular barbecued turkey legs. Some people attend fairs just for the food.

When my kids were young, the carnival at the county fair was in the front of their minds from the time it first showed on TV commercials during summer until we took them in September when it was finally open. These traveling shows were a bit scary to adults, especially the carnies working the rides and booths, but the kids always had a blast, getting on as many amusement park rides as we could afford.

If you don't mind neighbors, animals, walking or high-calorie food, there isn't much that is more enjoyable than a day at the fair. I highly recommend it!

=================

It just so happens that Roger Miller wrote a song or two about country fairs. My ending quote is from one such song, The Tom Green County Fair: "*Well, a Sunday at the fair can make a memory more valuable than gold, especially when you're 10 years old.*"

17. Glorious Sunsets

Previously, I had written about sunrises and how they are different from sunsets, and they are. Sunrises tend to be more brilliant than their evening counterparts, but typically don't come close to number and variety of shades and hues than the equivalent sunsets. By "equivalent," I mean that the weather and landscape allow the best view possible for both scenes, morning or evening. In many locations in the country, mountains and forest can completely obscure sunsets from view, as can heavy clouds, precipitation and other weather-related phenomena. Ironically, some clouds make both sunrises and sunsets much more dramatic than clear skies.

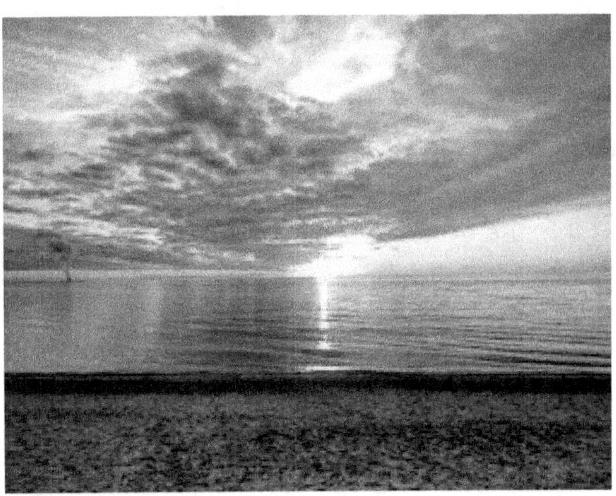

But, let's be honest. Glorious sunsets can be so moving as to deserve their own happiness category. I would compare sunsets with rainbows, which can have a spiritual effect on those who are fortunate enough to observe them, especially following extreme weather or rainstorms. When conditions are right and the ability to stop and gaze is present, it can be an awe-inspiring experience.

Colorful sunsets happen when the sun dips toward the horizon and its light has to travel through a greater distance of atmosphere before reaching our eyes. In so doing, blue light, as well as some green and yellow light, gets filtered out, leaving reds and oranges to continue in their place, and we can enjoy an abundance of those hues. Just about the only time you can see a red or orange sky is during a glorious sunset.

Like rainbows, which have been considered through the ages as a renewal or peace after tumultuous times, sunsets can symbolize the same at the end of a long day. They can represent the passage of time, the beauty of life and nature, and even the promise of romance. As the sun sets, light fades, which is symbolic of the forces of darkness.

I especially love sunsets beyond bodies of water, like the ocean or large lake, and am usually excited at that prospect when we arrive in such a location. One of the few disappointments of camping in the forest is that sunsets are almost certain to avoid us, just beyond the mountains and tree canopies.

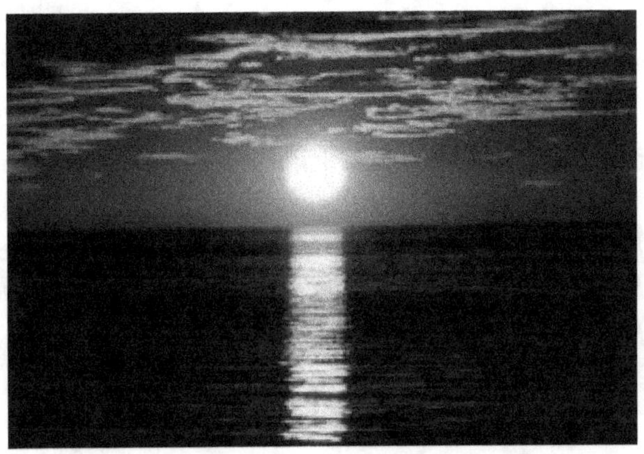

Let's not forget, when comparing to sunrises, that we are far more likely to be up and awake for a sunset. Especially in the summer months, sunrises are seriously ahead of my usual wake-up hour, making it a chore to see them, even with a good plan. However, I'm nearly always awake and ready for a dusk-time show.

Probably the best thing about a sunset, though, is the sheer surprise of the spectacle. No matter how many you may have seen over your lifetime, a beautiful sunset can seem like a miracle or an epiphany. The more glorious the view, the more astonishing it seems. I read a conversation online about how some people look to predict the best sunsets for planning the best time and place for viewing. This seems counterproductive to me, unless I am trying for sunset photos, for the surprise of the show is as awe-inspiring as the show itself.

=================

I'll leave the subject with some words from pop and Gospel singer/musician Amy Grant, who said, *"Get outside. Watch the sunrise. Watch the sunset. How does that make you feel? Does it make you feel big or tiny? Because there's something good about feeling both."*

18. Chocolate

Devil's food cake with dark chocolate frosting -- that's my all-time favorite dessert. Like most people, I've had a love affair with the cocoa bean as long as I can remember. Why do we love chocolate so?

Quora.com explains it this way: "The basic fact that chocolate tastes good and we enjoy eating it means that the body releases dopamine during chocolate consumption. ... Chocolate also contains theobromine, a chemical known to increase heart rate and energy, as well as arousal." Dopamine is the same chemical our brains release during sex, an adventurous experience or an especially gregarious laugh. Enough said.

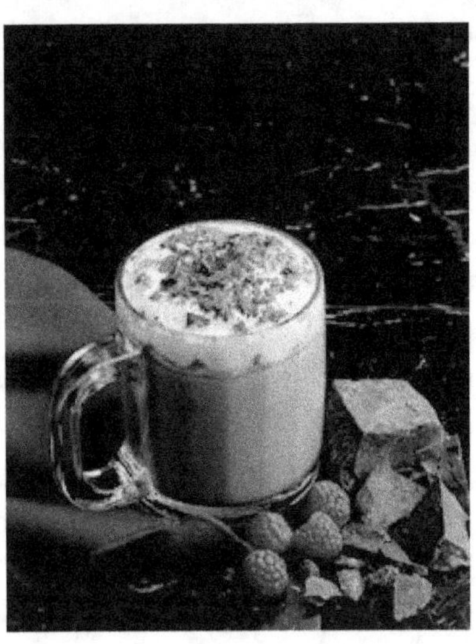

Lovers give chocolate when jewelry just won't do. According to History.com, almost 60 million pounds of chocolate are purchased in the U.S. during Valentine's Day week, proving an instinctual knowledge that the treat is a very successful way to someone's heart. Rich chocolate pairs with red wine splendidly, each enhancing the other and bringing an almost euphoric reaction to the taste. For good reason, a box of chocolates ("You never know what you're going to get.") is a staple for any husband in the doghouse. Only chocolate or chocolate chip cookie dough ice cream will do for binging after a break-up. Attend any convention's social hour and watch the crowd gather around the chocolate fountain with glee.

As much as you might like chocolate, it might be satisfying to know that there are a multitude of health benefits to indulging. Studies have shown that the flavonoids in chocolate can help keep your veins and arteries supple. Results also showed that participants in studies who were given several helpings of dark chocolate each week had significantly lowered their risk of heart attacks and strokes. One study even showed a lower risk of severe sunburn! Flavanols in hot cocoa provided an increased flow of blood to the brain and improved math skills. Subjects given bars of dark chocolate were shown to have overall lower LDL cholesterol levels. One extract from cocoa, lavado, can actually reduce the damage done to vital pathways to the brain by Alzheimer's disease. Chocolate can help to lower your blood pressure and increase endorphins, thereby helping prevent depression and other mental disorders.

It's been proven that white chocolate does not affect the brain the same as its brown counterpart and that you generally don't crave sweeter chocolate more than other types. In fact, chocolate that is less sweet also has less calories, and dark, smooth, melt-in-your-mouth chocolate can change your outlook on your whole day. We also know that having a small portion of dark chocolate can reduce food cravings, potentially saving you from binging on higher calorie treats.

I believe that if Hershey, Ghirardelli and Mars were to all shut down at once, no pandemic could match our collective reaction. Congress would act immediately to stem the crisis and the President would sign whatever bill he or she was presented, partisan politics be damned.

=================

My ending quote for this topic comes from British comedian Tommy Cooper: "*My wife said, 'Take me in your arms and whisper something soft and sweet.' I said, 'chocolate fudge.'*"

19. Photographs

The word "photography" comes from the Greek phrase "Drawing the Light." We all know that photography in the 19th century was cumbersome and time-consuming, and required technicians trained in the art form. But the photograms and photographs taken in those decades have provided an incredible and invaluable window into life back then. Color photos began to be produced by the mid-1880s and the first widely used color process hit the market in 1907.

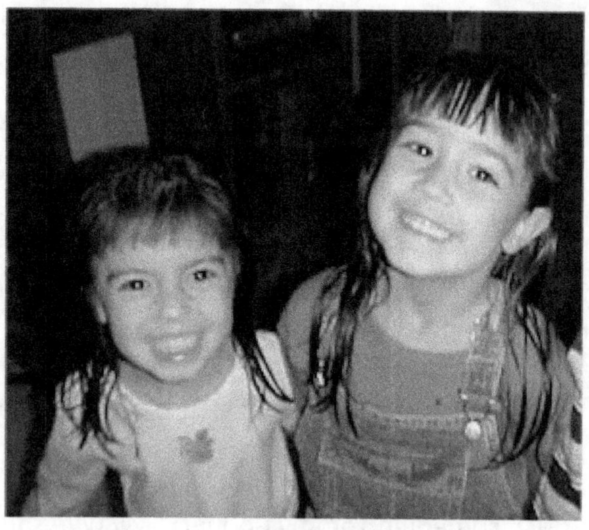

When cameras were developed that used roll film, photography became more widespread and amateurs were able to experience the joy of the hobby. Some were good enough or wealthy enough to go pro, which required more elaborate and expensive equipment. That's still somewhat true today, with the biggest difference between talented amateurs and professional photojournalists being the cost of their camera ensemble. Of course, today nobody uses film. For the younger readers, film was a medium, usually on a roll, that was placed inside of the camera, which was subjected to the light through the camera lens to produce either a film negative or slide positive image. Film then had to be developed by being taken to a film lab or, for a fortunate few, handled in their own lab, to produce paper photographs. Now, digital photography is the sole media everywhere — cameras, phones, watches, tablets, even dashboards in cars and trucks.

Photographs, whether paper or digital, are both useful and delightful for documenting family history and events, but also for capturing memorable times and places and documenting a person's life from birth to death. It is also quite valuable in capturing moments in nature, often providing views few individuals would ever otherwise see. Landscapes, cityscapes, oceanscapes, and skyscapes make up an incredible library of earth-based galleries, and for the past 50 years, outer space has provided a plethora of planet shots and other scenes from the universe.

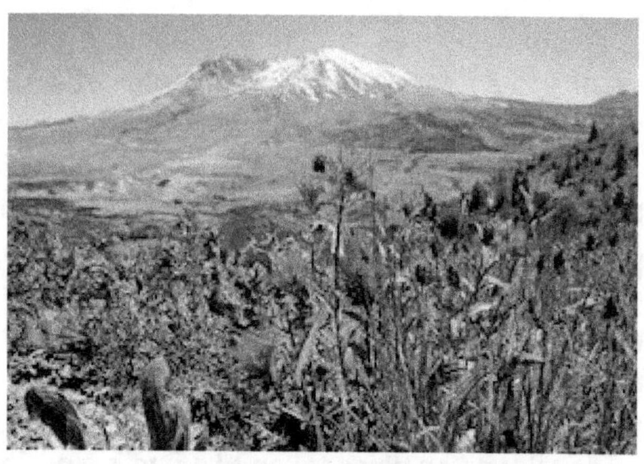

I once wrote a blog piece called, "In many ways, photos can offer more than video," about why I prefer still photos over video. In that article, I explain my opinion that video is spoon-fed to viewers, always making them focus on the movement and thinking about what the videographer intends. Photographs give a viewer time to think, time to explore the picture, time to remember similar sights, time to see what they can see and, more importantly, time to feel. Even though I've been recording video lately, I continue to feel it's true. A photographer also has more leeway to exclude and frame a shot. If you have ever seen a photo of a place you are familiar with, you might have had the feeling that the photo seemed more startling, colorful, insightful, clean or unusual than you remember. You experienced the photographer's eye.

My favorite photos? I love historic photography and magnificent landscapes, and I love to shoot abandoned buildings, birds, wildflowers, sunrises, sunsets and vivid shots of nature. I like family photos for their nostalgia, but still prefer nature.

=================

There is no one better to quote about photography than the ultimate landscape photographer and environmentalist, Ansel Adams: *"To photograph truthfully and effectively is to see beneath the surfaces and record the qualities of nature and humanity which live or are latent in all things."*

20. Gardening

When I was ten, we moved across the city to a house on a triangular lot with plenty of back yard. After I turned 12, I convinced my mom to let me take the far corner space behind a fence and grape vines, that was overgrown with weeds and the neighbor's ivy, and till it for a vegetable garden. I grabbed my brothers and a sister, ages 7 to 10, and we all went out and worked that dirt until it was clear and ready to plant, making sure we didn't disturb the old rhubarb plant. My mom told me to make raised rows to plant seeds in, leaving lower rows for watering, and we excitedly bought the seeds at the hardware store.

We planted radishes, zucchini, carrots, iceberg and green-leaf lettuce, bell peppers, sweet corn and pumpkins. The two weeks or so waiting for the first signs of growth felt like the week before Christmas -- like it would never arrive. When it finally did, all us kids kept it weeded and watered until we began harvesting our bounty. Did they ever taste great! A couple of months after the final veggies were taken, I was looking through the garden, reminiscing and planning for the next planting, I noticed something odd under the zucchini bushes. I reached down and pulled out the biggest zucchini I had ever seen, probably 2 feet long and 6 inches wide. Evidently every one of us had missed this one on our multiple picking sessions.

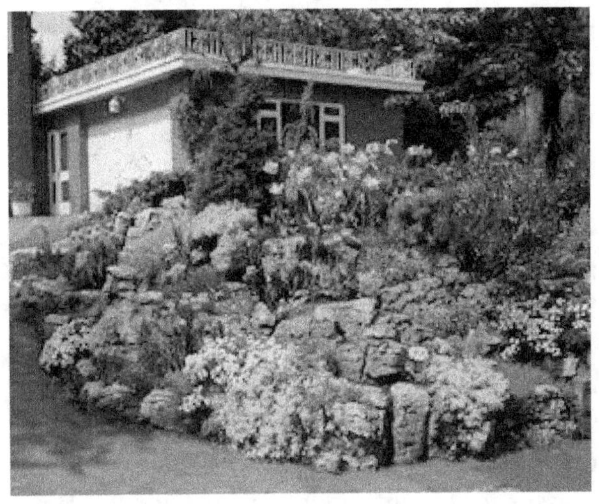

Outdoor gardening has many more benefits besides harvesting produce. Your skin actually turns sunlight into a nutrient, much like the plants you are working with. Vitamin D is essential for hundreds of body functions, including strengthening bones and your immune system, and can lower the risk of several cancers and multiple sclerosis. Low levels of vitamin D may increase the risk of several health conditions, including type II diabetes and dementia. Overexposure, however, puts you at greater risk of skin cancer, so you must either limit your sunshine or take other precautions.

Depending on the type of gardening you are participating in, various activities help exertion and exercise in several muscle groups, sometimes moderate to strenuous (like shoveling, digging or chopping wood), but even light exercise is beneficial. Gardening can also brighten your mood, help you recover from a depression or calm your body after a stressful event. Likewise if you are suffering from addiction.

Over the years I've lived in several houses, planted many a garden and grown dozens of fruit trees. The satisfaction of successful blooms and the birds, butterflies and hummingbirds they draw to us is like no other feeling. It is especially gratifying when you have selected the perfect mixture of colors, heights and duration of flowers, shrubs and grasses for the intended space. Even full-time on the road I put out feeders to draw birds to us, and, when we finally settle down in a home base, gardens will be cultivated.

=================

I'll end this topic with a quote from Alfred Austin, an English poet who lived at the turn of the 20th century: *"The glory of gardening: hands in the dirt, head in the sun, heart with nature. To nurture a garden is to feed not just the body, but the soul."*

21. The Internet

Hardly any waking moment goes by when I'm not using the Internet in some way. That got me to thinking about it, my 30+ years in IT notwithstanding. Life as we know it would not be possible without the Internet. First, a short history might be in order.

[Some of the following was paraphrased from Wikipedia.] Early packet switching networks [a "packet" of data is what computers use to communicate with each other and around a network] such as the NPL network, ARPANET, Merit Network and CYCLADES in the early 1970s researched and provided data networking. The ARPANET project and international working groups led to the development of protocols for inter-networking, in which multiple separate networks could be joined into a network of networks, which produced various standards. Research was published in 1973 that evolved into the Transmission Control Protocol (TCP) and Internet Protocol (IP), the two protocols of the Internet protocol suite. [You've probably seen "TCP/IP."]

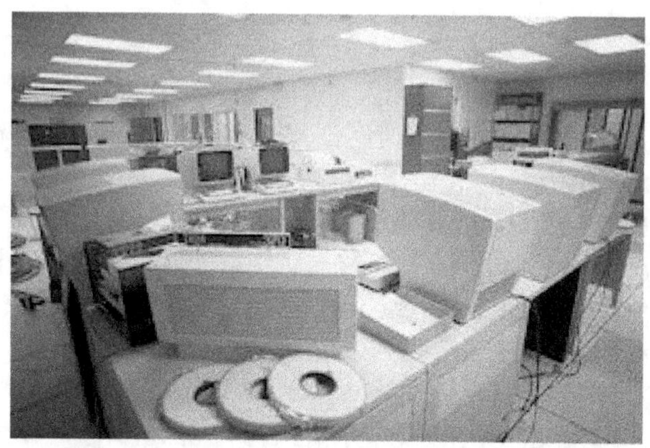

In the early 1980s the National Science Foundation funded national supercomputing centers at several universities in the United States and provided interconnectivity in 1986 with the NSFNET project, which created network access to these supercomputer sites for research and academic organizations in the United States. International connections to NSFNET, the emergence of architecture such as the Domain Name System, and the adoption of TCP/IP internationally marked the beginnings of the Internet.

Commercial Internet service providers (ISPs) began to emerge in the very late 1980s. The ARPANET was decommissioned in 1990 and the NSFNET was decommissioned in 1995, removing the last restrictions on the use of the Internet to carry commercial traffic. Commercial entities began marketing Internet access, content design, telephone and communications platforms, search engines and sales platforms. Facebook, Twitter, Google, YouTube, and all the other hugely successful web companies all owe that success to the National Science Foundation and ARPANET.

Today, the uses of the Internet are as numerous as the number of people on the planet. The top dozen most common uses, according to several reporting sites, are: email, research, downloading files, discussion groups, interactive games, education and self-improvement, movie/music/video streaming, friendship and dating, electronic newspapers and magazines, politicking, job hunting and shopping. Specific uses can be inferred from this list, such as virtual health appointments, maps and navigation, virtual meetings and teleconferencing, social media and long-distance family interactions.

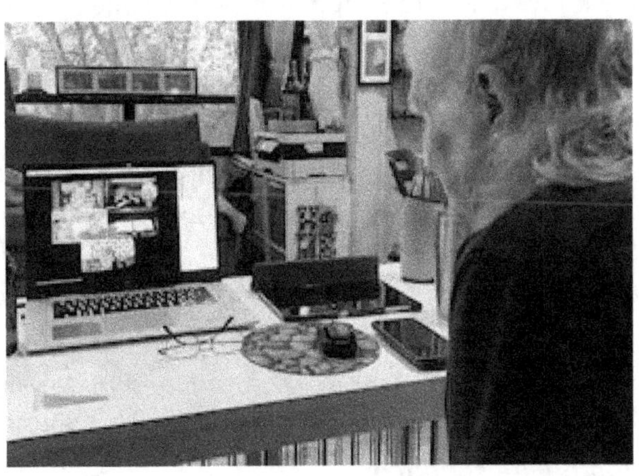

Like most people, there are times when I think the Internet is a pain, allowing anyone with a brain and access to spout any ideology they see fit, and the brain part may seem lacking. However, just maintaining long-distance family relationships can make all the difference in someone's life. The COVID-19 pandemic and the latest social injustice are two examples of events that bring us together utilizing the one communications service that seems to have been developed for just such occasions.

Would I be a published author without the Internet? Chances are slim. How easily could I share my 30,000 photos with the public? I've often referred to the Internet as my virtual memory, with nearly everything I would ever want to know at my fingertips. My blog would likely never have happened either, nor supplementing our income while living in an RV on the road. Like I said, life like we know it would simply not be possible.

==================

My closing quote for this subject is from Tom Wolfe, an American journalist, who said, "*Once you have speech, you don't have to wait for natural selection! If you want more strength, you build a stealth bomber; if you don't like bacteria, you invent penicillin; if you want to communicate faster, you invent the Internet. Once speech evolved, all of human life changed.*"

22. Back Roads

From the first moment I received my driver's license when I was a 16-year-old kid in Southern California, the back roads were calling me. Perhaps that was because of the crowded city life, or perhaps I longed to be free from the congestion of L.A. traffic. One thing was sure, once I took off for my first exploration of the Mojave Desert, I've always tried to avoid Interstates and major highways.

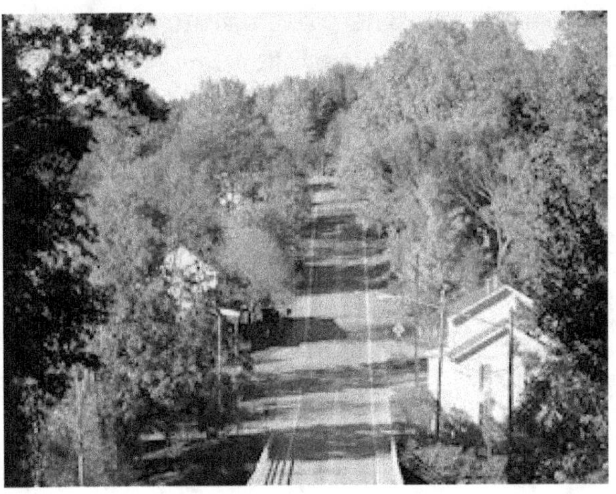

Now, freeways do have a great purpose -- they get you from point A to point B in the fastest time possible, even if some of that time is spent in bumper-to-bumper traffic. On a long trip, to completely avoid Interstates may add days to the journey, perhaps not a problem if you are retired, but definitely a consideration if just on vacation. You can always count on gas stations, truck stops and fast food, not to mention bathrooms, along a freeway or highway, not so much on the less-traveled roads. However, on the freeways, what you miss!

Dictionary.com defines a back road as "a little-used secondary road, especially one through a rural or sparsely populated area." The "rural" part is what makes it fun. From the forest roads of Colorado to the country hamlets of Upstate New York, from Texas' narrow "farm-to-market" routes to Oregon's scenic coastal byways, the pure pleasure of seeing nature, wildlife, country living, farmland and quaint Main Streets is totally absent from a jaunt on I-70 or I-95.

Certainly, half the fun of parking our fifth wheel in a new (for us) region of the country, even during the pandemic's "stay-in-place" orders, is exploring from our truck without any destination in mind (we often self-quarantined in the pickup), and our satellite navigation system almost completely ensures we won't get lost. The quirky "World's Largest" items in rural towns, the awe-inspiring fields of kinetic sculptures, the pure majesty of a redwood forest or a rugged coastline, the jaw-dropping views of the tallest jagged peaks, or a thunderstorm you can see 50 miles away, all of these things are experiences most likely missed on an Interstate highway. I take most of my photos of landscapes, wildlife, wildflowers and interesting rural scenes on these expeditions on back roads.

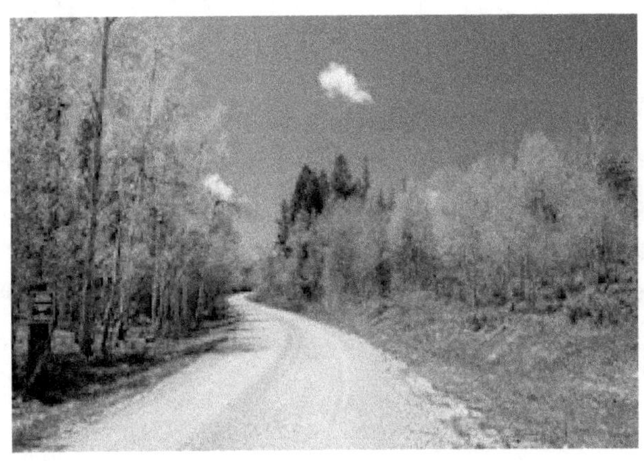

Something interesting to do, which we plan on attempting in the future, is to take U.S. Routes 66 and 20 from end to end. The famous Route 66 was one of the original highways in the U.S. Highway System and begins and ends in Santa Monica, Calif., to the west and Chicago, Ill., to the north. Most of us have been on parts of this historic highway already, but few have taken it from start to finish. Likewise, Route 20 is truly coast-to-coast, spanning 3,365 miles with endpoints in Boston, Mass., and Newport, Ore. Our living in Western New York gave us glimpses of this rural highway and we saw much of the western portion when we recently camped in Oregon. Both of these routes have been usurped in some sections by freeway, and it can be quite a task to try to stay on the original routes as much as possible, but even that process can be fun (if you like maps and navigation).

=================

My ending quote for this topic comes from Down Under, where Australian writer Robyn Davidson said, "*By taking to the road, we free ourselves of baggage, both physical and psychological. We walk back to our original condition, to our best selves.*"

23. Gadgets and Gizmos

A gadget, AKA gizmo, is defined by Dictionary.com as a "mechanical contrivance or device; any ingenious article." Ingenious seems to be the key word for making us happy.

A quick on-line search found just about as many articles about how technology and gadgets can make someone unhappy as there were for the happiness camp. I submit that if you view a gadget just as a tool to get something done, happiness might not even be considered in the equation. But, if a device is ingenious, the wonder and awe of it and its inventor can be euphoric. That's why so many tool sheds and kitchens are filled with gizmos and weird tools that may never be used. Before I became a full-time RVer, I was a member of that club. However, there's just no room in my fifth wheel for gadgets I won't ever use.

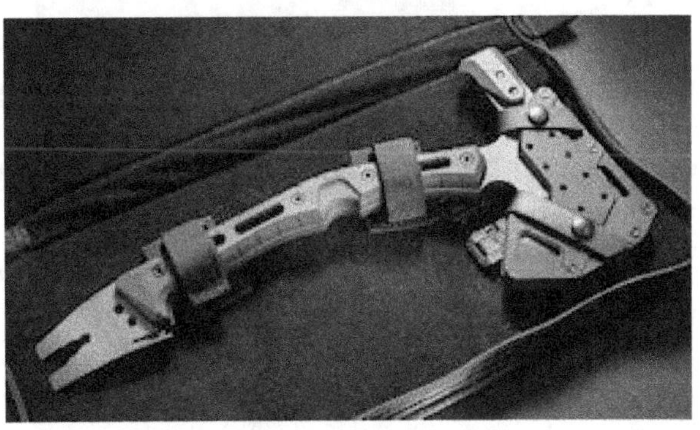

For myself, I keep a plastic miter box in my truck's tool cabinet because I never know when I might need to cut a piece of trim. I have actually used it three times in the two years we've been on the road. My other gadget pleasure is a tube of bungee straps of every size and shape. Interestingly, there are specialty straps made for specific tie-down solutions, such as for use with grommets in tarps and screens, with tent pegs and for multi-girth items. I love using them.

Gadgets have always intrigued movie-goers and TV fans, and Hollywood hasn't disappointed. Inspector Gadget, an animated series that began in 1983 and a 1999 movie, was a cyborg human with various bionic gadgets built into his body, though they often malfunctioned.

The polar opposite would have to be James Bond, who was given neat new gizmos by "Q" during each movie in the franchise, which nearly always proved to be useful or life-saving as the plot developed. The first Bond gadget was a Geiger counter, and that evolved to several versions of his briefcase, a phone-tap detector, a dagger-tipped shoe, a garrote wire and a laser cutting watch, homing beacons and pills, a miniature SCUBA set, in-air and underwater jetpacks, mini-rocket and cyanide cigarettes, cigarette guns, and so many more. It just wouldn't have been a 007 movie without them.

Science fiction has always had to develop new gadgets as visions of life in the future, such as the automatic doors in *Star Trek*, paper computers in *Mission Impossible*, spy contact lenses in *I Spy*, flying cars in *Blade Runner/Fifth Element/*hundreds of others, the neuralizer in *Men in Black*, *Back to the Future*'s hoverboard, and the ultimate gadget- the *Star Wars* lightsaber. I wouldn't mind having a few of these...

Innovation is almost always appreciated, but innovative gadgets always make you happy.

==================

As usual, I'll end this piece with a quote, this time from American writer Roger Zelazny: "*I have a fondness for technology. It's great to spend hours puttering around with mechanical things gotten from junkyards and visualizing what their use might be. Especially if you come across a gadget or tool and you don't know what it is and you try to figure it out. I'm fascinated by processes, whatever they might be.*"

24. Geocaching

Following a treasure map ... that is what geocaching is like, except the "X" that marks the spot is given in GPS coordinates and the treasure might just be the thrill of the hunt.

Wikipedia defines geocaching as "an outdoor recreational activity, in which participants use a Global Positioning System (GPS) receiver or mobile device and other navigational techniques to hide and seek containers, called "geocaches" or "caches," at specific locations marked by coordinates all over the world." Caches might be a large bin or lockbox, or a small coffee can, and "micro-caches" are often tiny pill bottles, matchboxes, spent bullet casings or plastic film containers. The contents, or "stash," usually consists of a small paper log and pencil for finders to check in and small trinkets, the odder the better. It has always been standard convention for seekers to take a trinket and leave one of their own, but many cache-hunters don't bother with either.

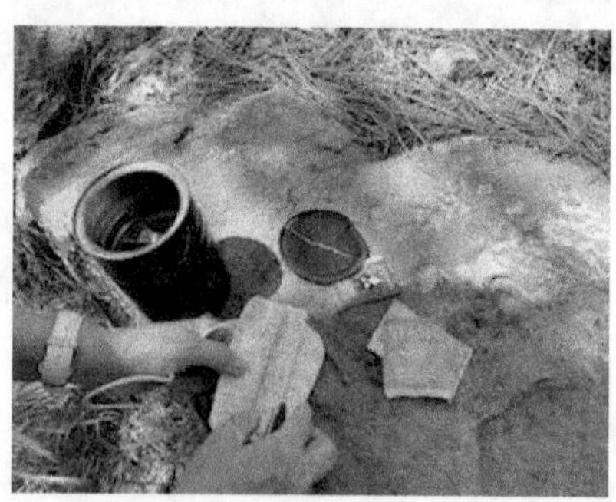

Whether you enjoy solving puzzles, treasure hunting, exploring, hiking or just being outdoors, geocaching is something you may love. In the days of social isolation, it can be an activity that brings much happiness. We have found caches hidden inside hollow tree trunks, hanging from tree branches, wedged between boulders, stuck on the side of a steel utility box and stuffed into a support pole of a culvert's guard rail.

You may have heard of the Fenn's Fortune, a hidden treasure of $1 million that wealthy art and antiquities dealer Forrest Fenn hid somewhere in the Rocky Mountain wilderness in 2010. He then published a poem of clues in his autobiography and treasure seekers have been hunting for the cache ever since. It has now been reported that the treasure chest was found in New Mexico (yes, the Rocky Mountains do stretch down into New Mexico). I bring up Fenn's treasure because clues are being used in geocaching more and more. You use the GPS coordinates to get close and then solving published clues or riddles helps you find the cache itself.

Cache hunters use popular websites and apps like Geocache.com or ExpertGPS (formerly GeoBuddy) to get a list of caches hidden in their vicinity, along with the GPS coordinates, otherwise people wouldn't know what was hidden in their area. These sites are used by the hiders as well so that seekers will be able to use their uploaded info to look for the stash. Once equipped with targets, hunters use their smartphones, GPS devices or car navigation to go to the coordinates. An included blurb normally gives a brief description of the cache and hints about where you might find it. Also important to us is how long it has been since the cache was last reported to be found. Weather, construction, vandals or other environmental influences can cause a cache to become missing completely, and the owner of the treasure might not know it yet. If something hasn't been reported found within the last year, we know chances are slim that we would find it in our own search.

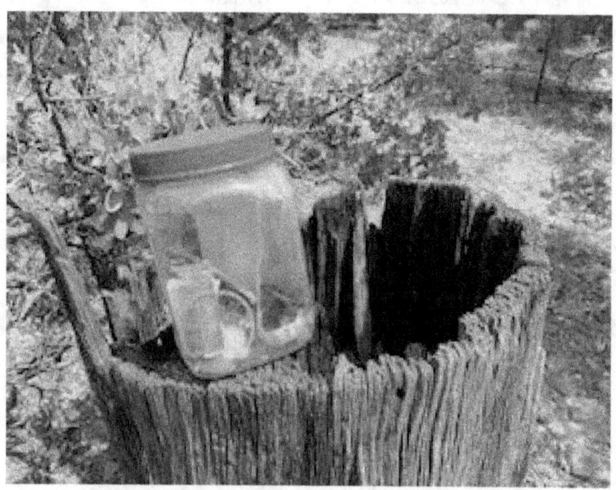

A few widely-accepted rules help the process. Most geocaching sites will not allow burying a cache and you must not hide one on private property unless it has free public access and you have permission from the property owners. Similarly, it should not be hidden in dangerous spots, like halfway up a steep incline, on a cliff or in the middle of a stream, and parking should be available somewhere nearby. Many of these cache containers are painted green, which is allowed, but it can make it difficult to find in a tree or bush, even if in plain sight. Popular sites and apps include a difficulty rating as well.

All of this so we can call out loud, "I found it!" No matter how frustrated we might get from failure, the next find more than makes up for it. Geocache hunting is also one of the few outdoor activities in which social distancing is built in. The search gets us outdoors and I often combine a photo shoot with the activity, doubling my enjoyment of the day.

=================

I'll finish with an oft-heard quote from frustrated cache seekers. "*I love it when the cache owner says that it's easy to find. Sure, it's easy for them. They hid it!*" —unknown

25. Sounds

Like smells, sounds can retrieve memories from long past or emotional times. A song played long ago at your wedding reception or at a parent's funeral service, a top-10 hit played on the radio during your high school years or a tune your mom or dad sang to you as a kid can each trigger thoughts of those scenes the moment you hear them. I'll be writing more about music in another topic.

Sounds can also be therapeutic. Sound and music therapy can help with meditation, relaxation and overall wellness. You might remember the "Sounds of Nature" displays at many department or grocery stores. I used to love to stand at the kiosk and listen to all the samples they offered. Similar therapies are also being used to combat a variety of ailments, including stress, anxiety, depression, high blood pressure, pain, high cholesterol, heart disease and risk of stroke. Even the hearing impaired can benefit from certain sound therapies through visual cues and "vibrotactile" feedback (listening to sound and music through vibrations in the body). After all, sound is a vibration that travels as an acoustic wave through a medium such as a gas, liquid or solid. It's the brain that translates the waves to a heard sound.

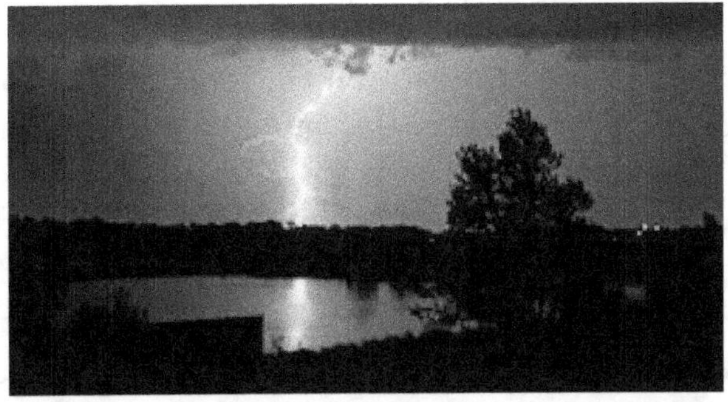

When I asked people what their favorite sound was, the most popular answers were what you might expect -- wind rustling through the trees, bird calls in the forest, babbling brooks and streams, crashing ocean waves and other of nature's reverberations. For myself, I would add a few different favorites. Many of the most awe-inspiring sounds I have experienced have indeed been from nature, such as a deafening clap from an approaching storm, a woodpecker hammering a tree in a forest, the freight-train roar of an approaching earthquake and the buzz of an almost invisible hummingbird zooming by. One of the more unusual came from deep inside a glacier in Alaska as a crack in the ice boomed thunderously in the bay toward us, 100 yards away. It reminded me of a frozen lake I was fishing on once as the sunshine began forcing the ice to crack from one shore to the other, only the glacial rumble was many times deeper in tone and more boisterous in force.

Even annoying noises can become part of your personal memory bank and hearing them again can result in pleasant reminiscing, such as the constant repercussion of a construction site you lived near during your first years in a relationship, or the din of a cattle ranch you visited as a child, or even traffic noise outside of your corner office window. Go to a zoo and the cacophony of calls may send you back to a grade school field trip. A baby's cry may remind you of your first born, long before you had your parental act together.

The simple truth is that sounds can make you smile. That happiness may come from the pleasantness of the tones, the comfort of the harmonies or the memories they conjure.

=================

As a final note, so to speak, Austrian philosopher Rudolf Steiner astutely observed: "*All of nature begins to whisper its secrets to us through its sounds. Sounds that were previously incomprehensible to our soul now become the meaningful language of nature.*"

26. Trees

Trees have been a wonderful gift to humans and the planet. Fossil records indicate that the first trees lived approximately 385 million years ago and they continued to flourish until they covered the earth as recently as 2 million years ago. They grow larger than shrubs and have a single main stem, but there is no defining attribute between a tree and a shrub, made more confusing by the existence of dwarf or small trees, and sometimes a tree's growth can be stunted by its environment.

By all estimations, there are over 3 trillion trees growing today, important for their value to the world: absorbing carbon dioxide, removing and storing the carbon while releasing oxygen back into the air, supplying wood for burning (for heat, cooking, creating power, etc.), giving timber for construction, providing shade for cooling, slowing water evaporation, providing food for humans and wildlife, and furnishing a canopy and habitat for wildlife, in addition to adding beauty with the seasonal changing of colors, brilliant flowers and leaves. It's pretty difficult to put up a kid's swing without a hefty tree branch to hang it from. Even forest fires can be beneficial -- killing disease and numerous insects that will prey on the growth of the forest, providing nutrients for new generations of growth and refreshing the various habitat zones the forest encompasses.

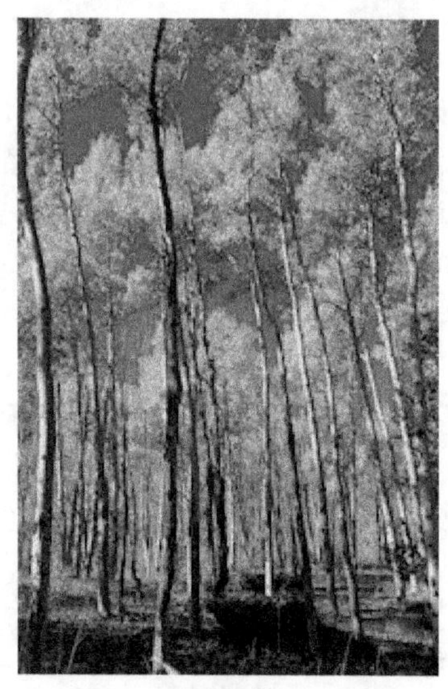

The largest, tallest and oldest trees in the world all happen to be located in California and Nevada, with the General Sherman Tree, a giant sequoia in Sequoia National Park, the largest by volume (52,500 cubic feet), Hyperion, a coastal redwood in Redwood National Park, the tallest (380 feet), and Promethius, a Great Basin bristlecone pine growing on Nevada's Wheeler Peak, the oldest (currently estimated to be 5,069 years old). An honorary mention goes to Methuselah, a bristlecone pine in California's Inyo National Forest, has a verified age of 4,852 years old.

While all of this is interesting, as well as important to humans' well-being, I compare a forest to the vivid draperies in an otherwise bleak apartment. Trees provide the backdrop to our views of the world and landscapes without them are often cold, somber or grim. Fall colors differ around the lower 48, with the yellows and light greens of the Rocky Mountains, the oranges and reds of New England and the full spectrum in the country's midsection. All are beautiful, sometimes spectacularly so, and we always look forward to drives through the colorful foliage in autumn, no matter where we happen to be.

Aspects and parts of a tree are often compared to human attributes, such as the roots, trunk, branches, growth, leaves and seeds. Having deep roots, a sturdy trunk, virtuous family branches, solid growth, spreading leaves of goodwill and the seeds of liberty are all positive expressions of humanity. Perhaps that is why the Japanese art of "bonsai" attempts to produce small trees that mimic the shape of real-life trees.

==================

The ever-famous naturalist and environmentalist John Muir, whose black-and-white photography of nature, true masterpieces, can profoundly move anyone who sees them, said, "*A few minutes ago every tree was excited, bowing to the roaring storm, waving, swirling, tossing their branches in glorious enthusiasm like worship. But though to the outer ear these trees are now silent, their songs never cease.*"

27. Air Conditioning

The early need for air conditioning grew out of the need to preserve foods, as those that are kept at room temperature spoil easily due to the growth of bacteria. At temperatures below 40 degrees, the growth of bacteria is reduced or eliminated. With the development of food refrigeration came air conditioning and humidity control shortly thereafter. The invention of absorption-type refrigeration in the early 19th century showed that liquefied ammonia could chill air when it is allowed to evaporate. Ice was created using compressor technology in the year 1842 by a physician named John Gorrie.

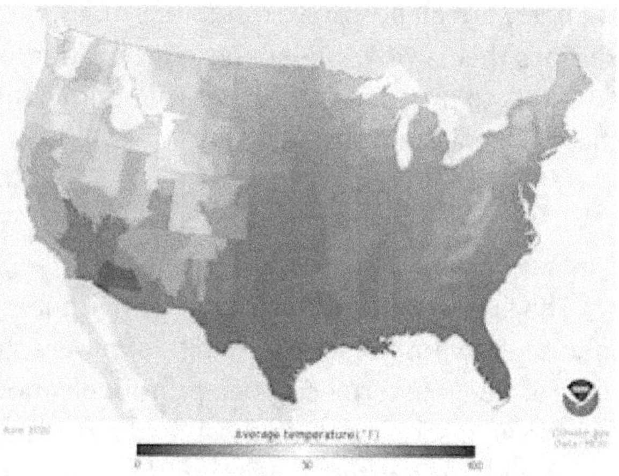

The first commercially-available air conditioning systems were used to cool air for industrial processes, rather than for personal comfort. The first electrical air conditioning was invented by Willis Carrier, the "Father of Modern Air Conditioning," in the year 1902. The rest, as they say, is history.

In America, hot temps begin, on average, in May for the southwest and in July for the rest of the country. Indeed, recently CNN reported, "A record-breaking heat wave is sweeping across the United States, and close to 90 percent of the population will experience 90-degree heat over the next seven days." So, you can see that air cooling is a must in much of the country.

I grew up in dry Southern California, so dry, in fact, that we had a giant evaporation cooler (AKA swamp cooler) that worked well. When I moved north to a more humid climate, I realized how good I had had it. Swamp coolers don't work well in high-humidity environments. In every place I have lived since my Washington State home, I have insisted upon air conditioning, which handles humidity as well as heat, including New York State, Nevada, Kansas and Colorado. Even in the desert of Las Vegas and the usually-dry elevation of Denver, summer monsoons can make the heat unbearable and swamp coolers ineffective. New York State and surrounding areas have wide swaths of homes without air conditioning. Apparently, the cost of installing the cooling systems far outweigh the relatively few seasonally hot days that it would be needed, so they sweat it out a few days every summer.

We now have A/C in our cars, trucks, RVs, supermarkets, schools and at most workplaces, and none of us can imagine life without it. There is nothing better than to come inside from a hard afternoon of working in the yard under a hot sun and sit on a cool sofa, preferably with the cold air blowing right at us. From what I can tell, A/C is one of the most underrated unsung heroes of 20th- and 21st-century living, allowing us to enjoy summer life instead of sweltering in it.

==================

Like myself, Bill Bryson is an American author who precedes modern air conditioning. He wrote, "*I grew up, really, in the days before air conditioning. So I can remember what it was like to be really hot, for instance, and I can remember what it was like when your barber shop and your local stores weren't air conditioned, so it was hot when you went in them and they propped the doors open.*"

28. The Ocean

I remember going to the beach as a kid growing up in Southern California. I have very fair skin and usually sunburned before I was enjoying the sand and waves for very long. After a few summers, I became proficient at building sand castles, skim surfing and surf Frisbee, and as a teen I would head to the piers as often as I could to fish for bonito. That wasn't very often.

The last time I visited Long Beach while I still lived in the Los Angeles area, it clouded up and a curtain of lightning bolts appeared on the sea's horizon. That storm closed in pretty quickly and I shot to my car and raced the thunderstorm home. The lightning and I arrived at the same time, with bolts striking towers and trees all around me. It was terrifying, but I did get to see ball lightning for the first and only time in my life.

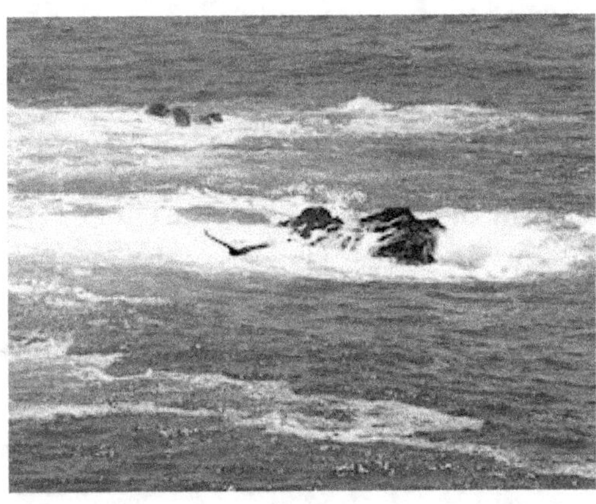

The oceans were created, according to current scientific thinking, millions of years ago by the escape of water vapor and other gases from volcanoes and the molten rocks of the Earth into the atmosphere, surrounding the cooling planet. Adding to this condensation was water and ice delivered by asteroids and comets over centuries or millennia. Without these phenomena, it is unlikely life would have formed on earth, and we wouldn't be here to explore its origins.

According to NOAA, the ocean produces over half of the world's oxygen and absorbs 50 times more carbon dioxide than our atmosphere. It transports heat from the equator to the poles, regulating our climate and weather patterns. From fishing to boating to kayaking and whale watching, the ocean provides us with many unique recreational activities. The world's oceans provide more than just seafood, with ingredients from the sea found in foods such as peanut butter and soymilk. Many medicinal products come from the ocean, including ingredients that help fight cancer, arthritis, Alzheimer's disease and heart disease.

Oh, but the waves! Waves are most commonly caused by wind. We have all seen cresting waves during a wind storm over a large lake or ocean, and this happens continuously somewhere in whatever vicinity you are located. Waves can also be caused by the gravitational pull of the moon and the sun (tides), by a weather or land disturbance off shore, such as during a hurricane or after an earthquake (tsunamis), or with large ships or land masses pushing the ocean ahead of them.

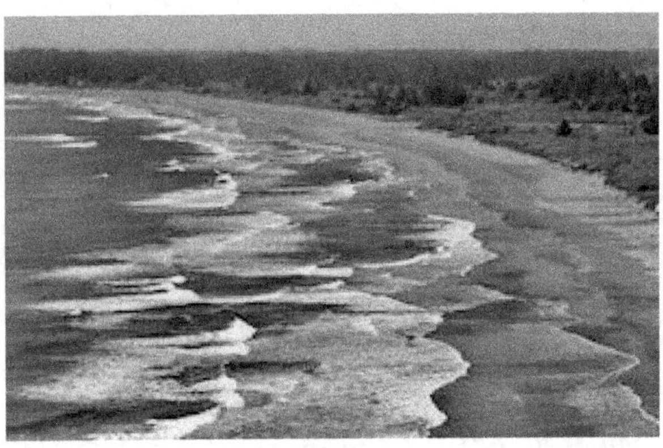

Research shows that those who live in homes by the coast experience better physical and mental health than those who do not. Homes with ocean views had even more positive results, with those residents feeling calmer than others. So, it's no wonder Hawaii ranked first by several Gallup polls as the happiest state in the U.S. The color blue is calming, and the constant ebb and flow you can both see and hear tends to be de-stimulating to your brain.

There is a long, detailed explanation as to why we have crashing waves at our shoreline, including orbital motion of the ocean's kinetic energy, but I find the mystery and wonder more appealing than the minutia. One need only stand on the beach or a cliff's edge for a few seconds watching nature's magic to get lost in it. The combination of the rhythmic pounding of the waves on the shore and the cadence of its crashing sounds, along with a continual rumble of all of the shoreline waves together, can sooth one's soul.

=================

Here is an interesting quote from 17th-century mathematician, Sir Isaac Newton: "*I do not know what I may appear to the world, but to myself I seem to have been only like a boy playing on the seashore, and diverting myself in now and then finding a smoother pebble or a prettier shell than ordinary, whilst the great ocean of truth lay all undiscovered before me.*"

29. Four Seasons

The Four Seasons was an American rock and pop band that became internationally successful in the '60s and '70s ... Just kidding. This is about the earth and its changing seasons.

Most people know that the four seasons -- spring, summer, autumn and winter — exist on earth as a result of its tilt on its axis, compared to its orbit around the sun. Knowing that the orbit is not perfectly round might cause one to think that summer happens when the earth is closest to the sun and winter when it's farthest away, but that is not the case.

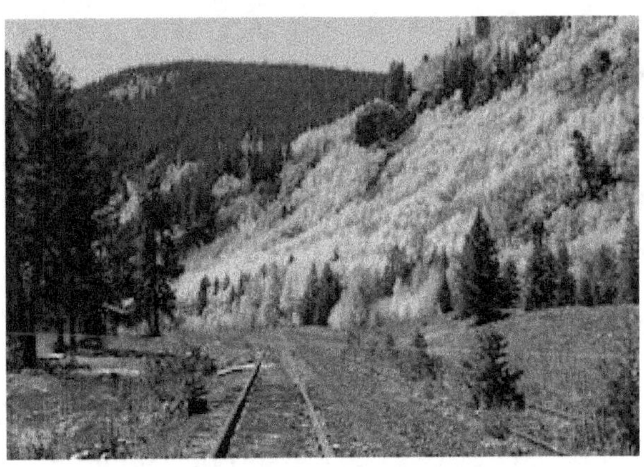

Because of the tilt, part of the earth is getting more energy from the sun in summer and less in winter. In spring and autumn, the amount of energy becomes more-or-less equal around the globe.

Also, because of the tilt, the northern and southern hemispheres enjoy opposite seasons from the other (the U.S. experiences summer while it is winter in Australia, and vice-versa).

But nature is not content to simply make the temperatures shift from one season to the next. The earth's climate revolves around the changes in solar energy, and each geologic region has its own peculiarities. Some are universal, such as snow and ice in winter, autumn changing of colors of leaves as the deciduous trees make less and less chlorophyll, flowers blooming in the spring and summer, and monsoons and hurricanes appear as the heat of summer warms the atmosphere and oceans.

Humans have adapted well to the seasons, especially in agriculture. This has enhanced hopes and expectations as each season begins to wane and make way for the next. Spring is for planting, and fall is forever harvest time. Summer is for work and play, while winter is for hunkering down and hibernation.

I have had the opportunity to live in a variety of locations around the country throughout my life, from the two seasons of California (summer and fall) to the two seasons of Western New York ("winter and August 12th," or "winter and construction," depending on who you ask), but also the four seasons in Washington State and Kansas. Even those areas that seem to skip seasons truthfully don't. You just have to be paying more attention.

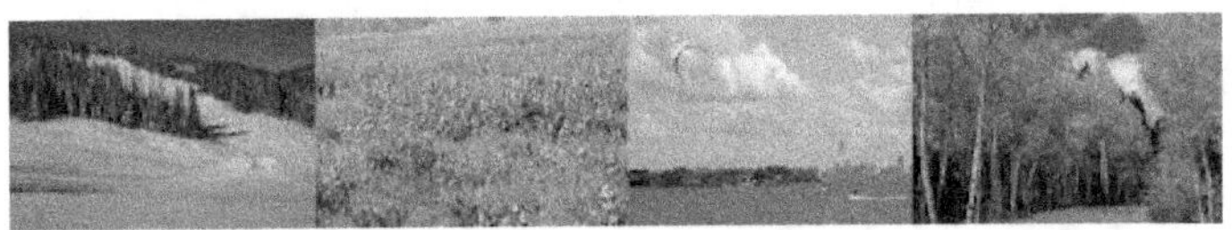

Contrast is a big reason that the changing seasons enhance the human experience. The warmth of spring and summer can be fully appreciated once one has survived the colder fall and winter. The rains of spring follow the snow or ice of winter. The heat of summer replaces the chill of spring. The cooler breezes and autumn storms follow the dry heat of summer.   The passage of time and of life is often chronicled with the change of one season to the next, or at least the passage is more felt.

As one would expect, everyone seems to have their own favorite and disliked seasons. Growing up in heat or cold doesn't necessarily make one like them more or less. It really is an individual taste. But, the universal themes of hope and anticipation accompany nearly every change of season. In my case, however, dread of winter was always my autumn emotion.

==================

I'll finish this discussion with a quote from American writer Rebecca Solnit, who said, "*For millions of years, this world has been a great gift to nearly everything living on it, a planet whose atmosphere, temperature, air, water, seasons and weather were precisely calibrated to allow us - the big us, including forests and oceans, species large and small - to flourish.*"

30. Holidays

When I was a kid, especially growing up the eldest of seven siblings, holidays were the stepping stones of happiness through each year. As soon as one was celebrated, we immediately looked forward to the next one. My grandparents held huge family 4th of July, Thanksgiving and Christmas parties and dinners every year, and I attended all of them until I was 17.

When I had my own kids, two of whom were born on Halloween (three years apart), I continued the tradition of celebrating as often as holidays came upon us. It was especially nice when they were a national holiday, meaning I could get an extra day off to stay with my family. Yes, Halloweens were extra-special in our house, with us usually have a double-birthday party with lots of their friends.

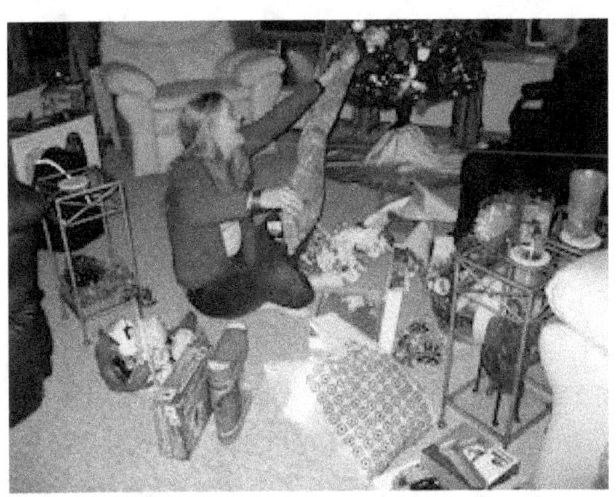

My kids grew up and I remarried, and with great distance between me and my kids and relatives, holidays became more of a meaningless chore than a reason to celebrate. It stopped making sense for Nadyne and me to give each other presents for birthdays or Christmas, since we usually bought whatever we wanted without waiting for a holiday or other excuse to do it. Besides, she was spending our money on me and I was spending our money on her. Holidays, other than getting time off work, stopped having the importance they had when there were children around.

Now that we are retired and not working, holidays are back to being happy stepping stones through the years, though without the excitement they once evoked. Being on the road, we love to visit all of our family members, wherever they are, but don't necessarily wait for holidays to do so. It's more about the geographical timing of our schedule. Independence Day fireworks at a son's house or birthday dinner with a daughter are always something to look forward to.

As a young adult, I enjoyed watching classic movies. *Holiday Inn* (1942, with Bing Crosby, Fred Astaire and Marjorie Reynolds with music by Irving Berlin) became one of my favorites. This is about a quaint Connecticut inn that some popular show business stars buy and hold holiday performances in. This is the first venue in which Bing Crosby sang

White Christmas, and it was so popular that it spawned his movie of the same name. I never miss Holiday Inn when this movie is on at Christmas time.

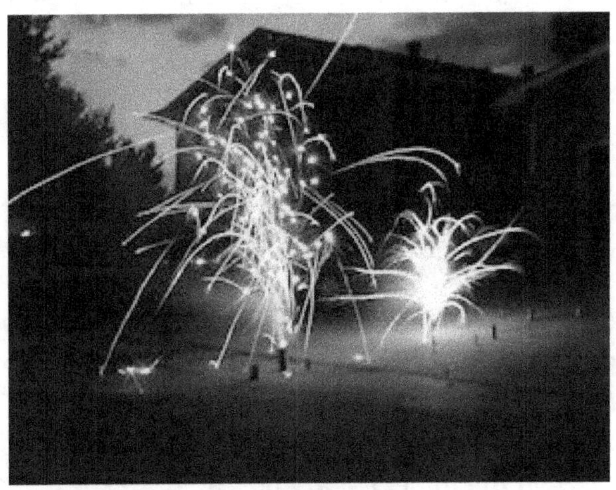

One thing about not getting caught up in the commercialism of each holiday is that we can enjoy the holiday itself. Also, we are happy to take advantage of seasonal sales for our own purposes. Why buy electronics in August when the Christmas season is around the corner?

One great thing about being in campgrounds during holidays is that campers are in a festive mood and are wanting to share good times with strangers. Many strangers become friends and we love to catch up with them as our itineraries cross. Thanksgiving in an RV resort can be wonderful!

Just as a sunrise can fill someone with hope and determination for the coming day, so can New Year's Day be a day of resolution to be better, with wishes for dreams and ambitions, and hope for humanity. After all, it's called "New Year's Day," not "Old Year's Passing Day."

==================

I'll finish this topic with a quote from Canadian actress Rachel McAdams, who said, "*I had a lovely childhood. For family holidays, we went as far as the car could take us - we would drive to Florida, even though it would take three days. I didn't know we didn't have a lot of money because there was always food on the table. I didn't have a lot of stuff, but I did figure skating for a long time, and I always had my skates.*"

31. Hiking Trails

My first hike occurred when I was in the Boy Scouts at age 14 in the Los Angeles area. My troop's leaders drove us up into the San Gabriel Mountains to a trail head and we proceeded to hike 6 miles up into the forest. I hated every minute of it.

We set up camp for the weekend and, on Sunday, we broke camp and hiked back down the trail — a bit easier walk, but I was still not a fan. I had overpacked, which wasn't ever going to happen again. A few months later, we hiked one of the Seven Peaks trails in the San Bernardino Mountains. That was the first time I had climbed to a mountain peak. Looking down over the valley below was exhilarating, despite poor visibility through the smog.

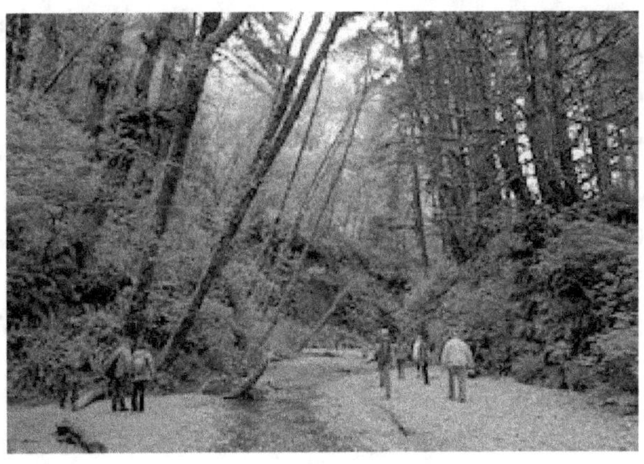

Health-wise, hiking is one of the best all-round activities you can do. Here are the Top 10 from Health Fitness Revolution and author of the book, "ReSYNC Your Life," Samir Becic: hiking increases fitness, allows you to take control of your workouts, tones the whole body, helps prevent and control diabetes, lowers blood pressure and cholesterol, and may improve the antioxidative capacity in the blood of oncological patients, helping to fight off the disease. It's a social activity that increases creativity, increases happiness levels, curbs depression and allows you to commune with nature.

My own preference for hiking really stems from my vagabond spirit -- there is only so much of nature to see from the highway. On one of my hikes in the mountains when I was in my 20s, about 5 miles from the road, we came across a car, probably circa 1920s, terribly rusted and nearly completely imbedded into the mound of dirt in which it was sitting. On another walk at Lake Mead, outside of Las Vegas, I found a dilapidated pleasure boat from the '50s or '60s sitting on the desert floor, in an area exposed from the lake's recent retreat due to drought. You just never know what you're going to see. Also, the farther you are from civilization, the more apt you are to witness wildlife — in the wild.

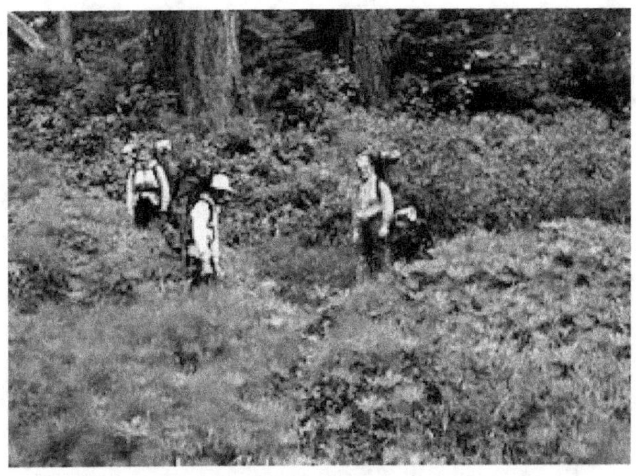

In America, we are so fortunate to have city, county, state and federal departments that create and maintain hiking trails in all 50 states. You can hike in so many terrains, too, including sandy desert, rocky mountains, thick forests, alpine elevations, spongy tundra, dripping wetlands, lake or ocean beaches, and so much more. Although public abuse of those trails has begun to force some trail closures or additional fees, there still seems to be a commitment by the appropriate agencies to keep lands available to use. Also, there are many volunteer groups that periodically tend to trails and trail heads.

==================

I'll end with a quote from American journalist Nicholas Kristof, who said, "*Wilderness trails constitute a rare space in America marked by economic diversity. Lawyers and construction workers get bitten by the same mosquitoes and sip from the same streams; there are none of the usual signals about socioeconomic status, for most hikers are in shorts and a T-shirt and enveloped by an aroma that would make a skunk queasy.*"

32. Online Repair Instruction

The first time I used the Internet to learn how to do a household repair was for a broken 37-inch LCD TV. It would have cost over $400 to repair in a shop, at the time more than half of the purchase of a new TV, which was usually at the top of my pain threshold. Since it was either repair it myself or throw it away, I really had nothing to lose. The problem had been that the TV would turn on and run for about a minute, then power off, no matter the video or power source. I went to YouTube and searched for the issue along with the TV's make and model and viola! There it was!

I watched the 15-minute video three times and became confident that they had accurately described the issue and the resolution. I opened up the back of the TV, which was difficult with 14 screws in odd places, and documented where the screws had come from. I located the board that was supposedly the problem and disconnected it. I then called a few TV repair shops that advertised that they sold parts and got quotes for the board as well as some confirmation that this was the issue. The new board only cost $59 and I picked it up from the shop when they called to say it was in, just about two weeks later. I installed the new circuit board and reassembled the TV (all but one screw, for which I couldn't find the spot), plugged it in and stood back. I pressed the power button on the remote and the TV's picture slowly appeared. About 10 anxious minutes later it was still on and running properly and I felt pretty good about myself. That TV went on for another two years before we gave it away when downsizing to move into our fifth wheel.

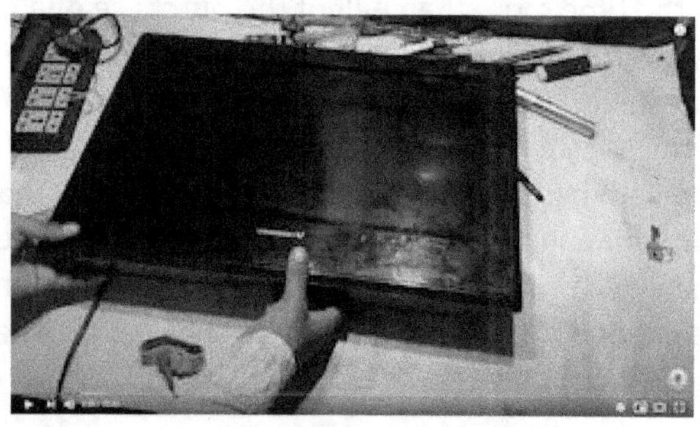

Many of us take the Internet for granted. I come from the BI era (Before Internet). I once owned a computer sales and repair shop and had five four-drawer file cabinets just to collect and store manuals and tech data for everything we sold or worked on. With each model update, we had to a) know about it, b) request info for it, and c) file the paper manuals and tech data we received, assuming we did. If we had an odd repair on something for which we didn't store specs or schematics, we would have to call the manufacturer, which could mean hours on hold before talking to someone who may or may not speak English well, and wait for the manual and repair instructions to come in the mail, or later, via email. If you were the unfortunate customer waiting for your essential equipment, it might have been quite a wait.

I remember when Seagate, one of the largest hard drive manufacturers in the country, placed all of their tech manuals online, right on their site, causing many a tech to have tears in their eyes. Western Digital soon followed, then Hewlett Packard, IBM and everyone else. Eventually consumer manufacturers caught up and put their manuals online, realizing that their own support volume would be reduced, which happened.

That is the technical specifications side of repairs, but you were still dependent upon technicians to diagnose and repair your equipment, and that wasn't always cost or time effective. Enter YouTube and the mighty geeks who decided to show off their skills. Repair videos became so popular that more and more types of content were created, including how-to, when-to and why-to videos for the RV and travel industry and for the millions of homeowners wanting to DIY.

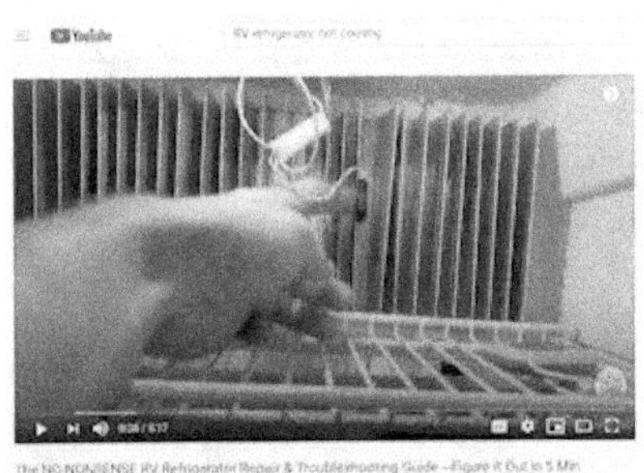
The NO-NONSENSE RV Refrigerator Repair & Troubleshooting Guide - Figure it Out in 5 Min

When I wanted to install my fifth wheel flooring, I watched videos on the various choices, selected one, and then several more videos on how to purchase and install it. It was a two-day job, but it turned out well and was a fraction of the cost of having a pro install it. When my awning switch went out, or my refrigerator stopped cooling, or my generator refused to start, the Internet came to my rescue, though I did decide to let a tech do some of those repairs. Each was an informed choice.

Other uses of this valuable resource include automotive and engine repair, hobbies (e.g., RC planes and drones), plumbing, gardening, birding, and on and on and on. I don't recommend doing electrical repairs yourself — obviously an electrician should be hired whenever possible — but that doesn't mean you shouldn't become an informed consumer beforehand.

=================

I take this quote by Apple CEO Tim Cook to heart. When speaking about online information, he said, "*We shouldn't all be fixated just on what's not available. We should take a step back and look at the total that's available, because there's a mountain of information about us.*"

33. Life Companions

Scientifically, men and women who commit to life-long relationships, regardless of the gender mix, not only live longer but have much happier and healthier lives than their single counterparts. This is especially true when times are dark, such as in a significant economic downturn or a public health crisis. It seems we all crave the support of a loved one to share pain, sorrow, elation, happiness and life experiences, good and bad.

Unfortunately, there are as many hits as misses when it comes to partnering with a soul mate. In a world of 8 billion people, there is no shortage of those who aren't "the one." A pessimist would see this as an impossible situation, especially if they believe there is only one perfect mate for someone. I don't believe that, but rather, as an optimist, that life is what you make of it. People who are somewhat compatible can make an even better couple than those who seem to be 100 percent compatible. Once a connection is made, the success of a couple can be a mixture of morals, temperament, respect, past experiences and openness to love. In my opinion, a majority of couples has what it takes.

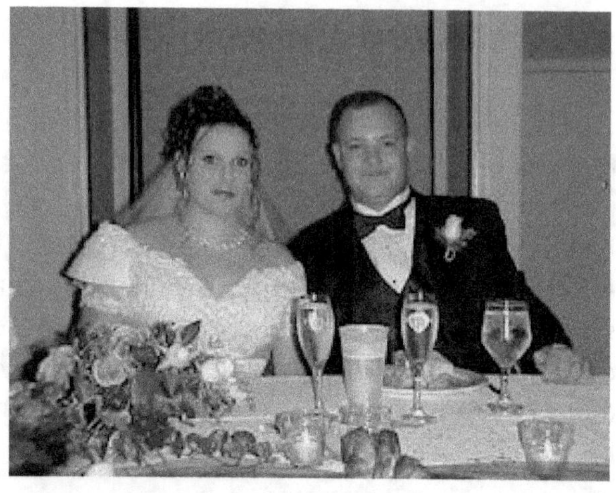

We all know those lovebirds who met as kids, married out of high school and were together their entire adult lives. For most of us, that is an impossible bar to reach, meaning that very few people meet their soulmate that early in life. Normally it takes time, effort, knowing oneself and being open to possibilities. I started out thinking I would be with my wife forever, then found out in just a few years that it was not going to be the case. After 26 years I divorced, then married my actual soulmate, and I was her third husband. That was over 20 years ago. We were across the country from each other but still managed to meet, fall in love and move in together. There is no rule of thumb when it comes to coupling.

Researchers have found that couples who are hostile to each other have more stress hormones in their systems and have generally less healthy lives.

Fortunately, the opposite is also true, which means that it is well worth any effort to be with a partner with whom you can enjoy life.

Happiness can be fleeting and you can't force it upon yourself. However, you can recognize when you experience it and rejoice in a life worth living. A spouse, significant other, a life partner, a POSSLQ, or however you want to define your committed partner, are one of the keys to a happy life. The tenet, "Happy wife, happy life," could really be used to describe any partner in a relationship. Most of the happy couples we know don't argue, they discuss respectively, the difference being that, in the latter, the need to win is missing. They, like us, want the best for their spouse or partner, and that is the priority.

According to Psychology Today, "Good relationships make people happy because a dependable companionship is a basic human need. Improving social relationships will bring our happiness score up. There is strong consensus in the field of positive psychology that the number and depth of personal relationships has the greatest effect of all on happiness. And the relationship where vast numbers of people derive that greatest boost to their well-being is in their marriage."

These benefits are valid in mixed race, gay, transgender and bisexual relationships, especially when the couples have strong support from their friends, families and co-workers. The LGBTQ community can provide a great social network for those couples needing additional support.

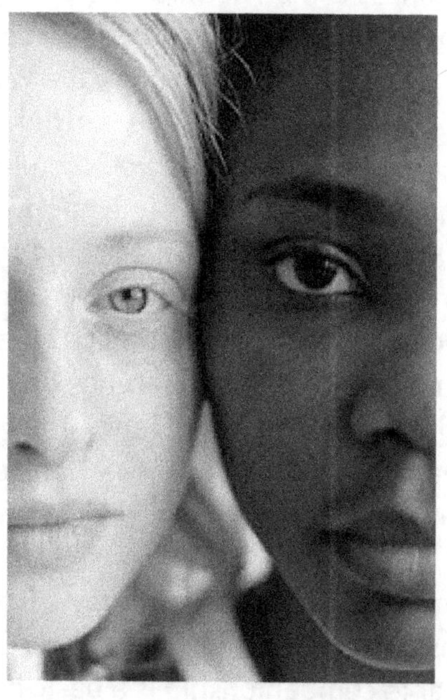

Watch any long-time couple and you may see a symphony of synchronicity. Each knows how to make the other feel good and they do so in little ways all the time, anticipating needs and accommodating as they can.

Another excerpt from the same Psychology Today column is, "Dependable companionship is a basic human need." There it is. When looking for things that make us happy, a companion is one of the most basic. Don't take it for granted and do the little things to nurture your relationship. Together, a couple can weather storms and enjoy life together so much better than individuals alone. Revel in it.

=================

I'll close with a quote from late English actor and entertainer Bruce Forsyth, who once said, "*The secret to a happy marriage is if you can be at peace with someone within four walls, if you are content because the one you love is near to you, either upstairs or downstairs, or in the same room, and you feel that warmth that you don't find very often, then that is what love is all about.*"

34. Picnic Lunches

Some of my earliest memories are picnic lunches at the neighborhood park with my mom and dad, along with my younger brothers and sisters. Dad always brought a kite and we would spend hours keeping it flying. Mom's lunches were always great.

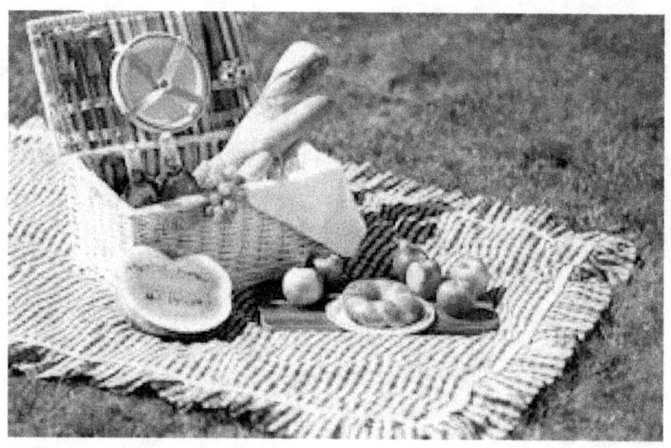

One of the great things about picnics is that there is no particular location necessary for them. You can enjoy a meal at the park, on a hike, during a drive or even on a rooftop. We almost always brought lunch from home when we went fishing and I'm certain hunters do the same, as do many cyclists, hikers, boaters and other outdoors enthusiasts. Popular locations besides the park include the mountains, the beach, in canyons, a forest, a lake, a fun place in your city, in a nearby city or town, your backyard, at summer concerts, at festivals or fairs, at sporting events and even the library. One of my favorite concert venues is in Washington State, the Gorge Amphitheater in George, in which half of the seating is on tiered grassy areas perfect for picnic lunches.

Being outdoors is itself a beneficial thing to do for your health, with sunshine, outside air, and beautiful vistas all contributing to your well-being. A jaunt into the wilderness can inspire, and a packed lunch will help you get even further away from civilization. Many health benefits do not require strenuous exercise, so a drive to a roadside picnic table on an overlook or in a national forest will still do some good.

The right setting and ambiance can facilitate romance, with many a first date made accordingly. Lots of games and sports are available to kids and adults alike during a day at the park, and an entire industry was built from what started out as weekend barbecues. Lifelong memories can be made and lifetime events such as birthdays, engagements and anniversaries can happen at picnics.

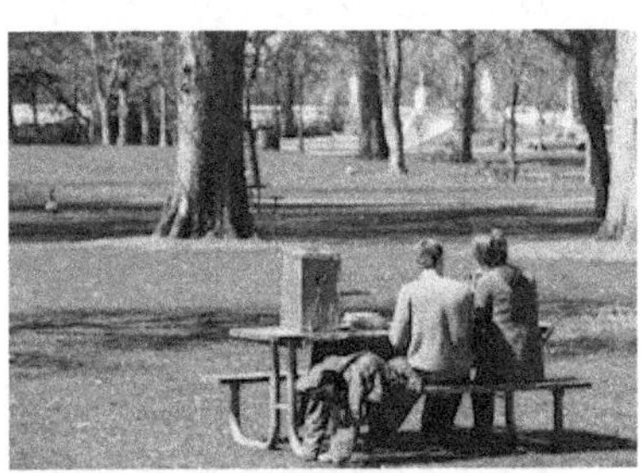

The tools of picnicking are those that nearly everyone uses, like picnic baskets, tablecloths, plasticware, drink jugs, paper or plastic cups and napkins or paper towels. That makes this activity one of the few widely shared activities around the world. A picnic lunch in the English countryside looks very similar to one in Central Park or near a French vineyard or on a Greek island. A Rocky Mountain lunch is comparable to one in the Italian Alps or Bavarian Black Forest or in the Andes, and a packed lunch in a Kansas wheat field is much the same as the meadows in England, though I might suggest you avoid picnicking on the Serengeti or in the Brazilian rainforest.

Last, a picnic will cost much less than a restaurant, and is far more secluded, so they continue to be as popular as ever.

==================

I'll end this discussion with an appropriate quote from English actress Kate Winslet, who said: "*The things that make me happiest in the whole world are going on the occasional picnic, either with my children or with my partner; big family gatherings; and being able to go to the grocery store - if I can get those things in, I'm doing good.*"

35. Baseball

"In a year that has been so improbable ... the impossible has happened!"

That was Vin Scully announcing Game 1 of the 1988 World Series, immediately following a famous bottom-of-the-ninth home run by a hobbling Kirk Gibson, batting against closer-extraordinaire Dennis Eckersley. The walk-off homer, as they now call them, won the game for the Los Angeles Dodgers and gave them the momentum needed to beat the Oakland A's for their last World Series title. I was 32 in October that year and remember that home run like it was yesterday. I was camping with my brother in a remote stretch of the Columbia River in Washington State and felt very fortunate to be able to receive the broadcast where we were. We were about 20 miles from the nearest town, but they may have heard us whoop and holler that night.

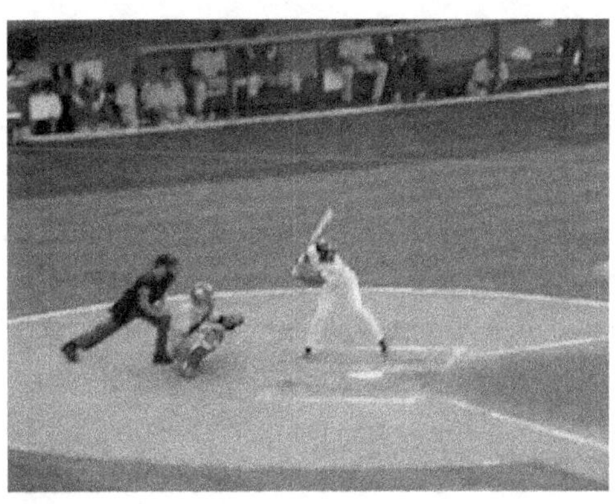

I grew up in the L.A. area and was a huge Dodger fan, but I would not have been as big a fan if I hadn't spent a lot of time in the playground playing baseball. There are several reasons why I think baseball is better for kids than other sports, but I had very good hand-eye coordination, could easily run, catch and hit, but, most importantly, it was one of the few sports in which my diminutive height as a kid didn't affect my skill and success. I did have asthma, so organized ball was out, but that didn't keep me from helping my best friend train in high school, and it didn't keep me from enjoying baseball on the school grounds. And I was pretty good.

Like golf, bowling, tennis, wrestling, volleyball, football, soccer and swimming, people who have played the sport are much more likely to watch them when they can't play. Baseball is also considered "America's National Pastime," which is a nod to its even wider appeal, similar to soccer and football, but it was the first truly national sport in the U.S.

Baseball is different from most other sports in that it doesn't have a time limit. A game can theoretically go on forever. When the pitcher has the baseball and there are runners on base or a tied score, intensity rises as he holds the ball. The longer he holds it, the more intensity that builds. I remember many times when the pitcher just didn't want to throw the ball, afraid of the outcome.

Occasionally the umpire would even have to step out to tell the pitcher to continue the game. Eventually, the pitcher does throw it, with or without the umpire's warning, once convinced that he must.

Baseball mimics life in a way. It runs on a serial timeline in which the life of the game literally follows the ball. It is more fair than real life in that both teams will always have the same number of opportunities for offense. A home run in the top of the 13th inning, for instance, doesn't automatically win the game, since the other team gets to have its at-bats in the bottom of the inning. If they tie the game, on to the 14th inning they go.

There have been so many exciting moments in this sport that's been played since the middle of the 19th century that you can write an encyclopedia-sized collection of them. (For younger readers, an encyclopedia used to be a set of dozens of books containing articles, history and a collection of all shared knowledge at the time of its printing.) Society's problems have been baseball's problems, too, and its social remedies have not always kept pace. Now it's a worldwide sport, with hundreds of foreign-born professional players in the major and minor leagues. But none of that would matter as much if I had never played it myself.

==================

My final quote is from Herbert Hoover, the 31st President of the U.S.: "*Next to religion, baseball has had a greater impact on our American way of life than any other American institution.*"

36. Ingenuity

Ingenuity is defined by Dictionary.com as "the quality of being cleverly inventive or resourceful." My own take is that proof of ingenuity can be seen in a solution to a problem or inconvenience that is not obvious to very many people. Think MacGyver, but scaled back.

As many an RVer will convey, problem solving without ready-to-use, off-the-shelf solutions is an integral part of the lifestyle. Those that can't do it need to have lots of time and cash.

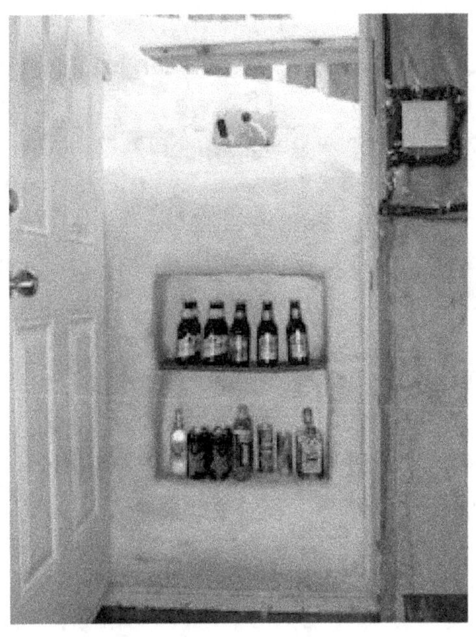

Here is an example: When we decided to upgrade our portable generator, the new unit wouldn't fit in the old storage spot. There was no room in the back of the pickup, since I had two large toolboxes installed in its bed, nor would it fit in any basement compartment in the fifth wheel. It was going to take a unique solution, one not readily apparent at first look.

I realized that there would be room on the rear bumper if I could find a way to attach a cabinet or shelf back there. Also, I had had the fifth wheel's original flimsy rear bumper replaced with a sturdy steel square pipe welded to the frame after experiencing problems with it, so weight on the bumper shouldn't have been an issue. We had previously had a dual bicycle rack clamped to the bumper when we had heavy electric bikes, and, when we sold the bikes, I kept the racks. When clamped tightly on the bumper, several people could stand on it without it sagging, so I guessed a wooden shelf would be stable.

I bought and cut 2-inch by 8-inch lumber and several lag bolts, washers and nuts, and, after applying several coats of waterproofing, attached the boards on the bike racks. I countersunk the tops of the bolts so they would not impede anything I placed on it. Once satisfied of weight-bearing success, I removed the back of a painted steel office cabinet and screwed it down on the shelf so as to not block the license plate. I had purchased a generator that would fit side-to-side through the locking cabinet doors, and secured it onto the cabinet floor and some boards I placed inside it just for that purpose. The doors close and lock, and though it wouldn't totally prevent someone from stealing it, it makes it difficult enough. With the rear of the cabinet completely removed, there is plenty of air circulation for the generator as well. The starting cord is easily available on the side and behind the cabinet, and the gas tank can be reached with a funnel just behind the top of the cabinet.

For good measure, I secured my 50-amp cord spooler down on the shelf, and now I have my pet fence sections strapped back there as well for easy access (instead of in my basement compartment).

I feel pretty good about my solution, which is just one example of a setup that took ingenuity and a bit of carpentry skill. Like I said, difficulties and clever answers are just a part of life on the road.

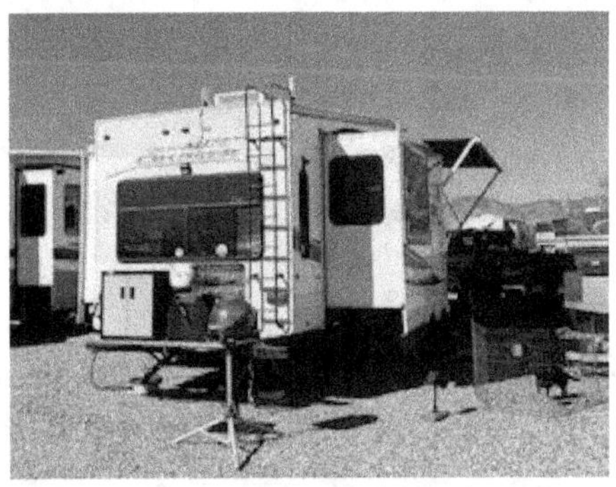

Nadyne has been equally ingenious on the inside of the rig. One problem we were having was with setup and tear-down between stays — in other words, before and after travel days. As all frequent travelers know, anything on a counter top in the rig tends to shift, vibrate and move while on the highway. It is very time consuming to secure all of these items for travel, strapping some down, placing some on the sofa or bed, and just all-around stuffing wherever they would fit snugly. It is even more time-consuming to set everything back up for use.

Museum gel works fine on smaller items like wine bottles and knick-knacks, but not so much on small appliances like our ice maker, coffee maker, air fryer, or other kitchen necessities such as silverware and plate caddies. She searched high and low for a solution with the common marketplaces apparently no help.

She remembered how sticky some rubber mats are and wondered if they would hold larger items. She bought a roll of rubber matting and cut some pieces just big enough for the aforementioned appliances and caddies to sit on. We left them in place on the counters on our next travel day, stopping occasionally to check for movement (or damage), and were pleasantly surprised how well things had stayed put on the mats. She found some rubberized cooking sheets that were less expensive but had the same gripping power. We stocked up, then started snipping and using them for other pieces of equipment around the rig, such as our laptops, adding machine, printer, alarm clock and even some electronics for the TV in the bedroom. Since doing that two years ago, we have not lost a single item off of any cabinet, desk or counter due to the road vibration and sway, even on the Pennsylvania Turnpike that was rough enough to break our rig's springs.

I would imagine if you ask any full-time RVer, they can regale you with wonderful stories of their own ingenuity. Aw, shucks...

==================

I'll finish this discussion with a thought from American author Shelby Steele, who said, "*We are a nation with a powerful investment in the idea of our own fundamental innocence. Our can-do optimism and ingenuity are based on the faith that we are a decent, open and generous people. This is our identity.*"

37. Dreams

Most dreams are forgotten by the time you wake up, let alone after. But that doesn't mean they aren't instrumental in a happy, healthy life. WebMD defines dreams as "basically stories and images that our mind creates while we sleep."

According to Medical News Today, there are 55 different themes or categories of dreams common to many people. Some of these are being chased or pursued, sexual experiences, falling, flying, arriving too late, a living person being dead, being nude or inappropriately dressed, being frozen with fright, racing or losing control of a vehicle, and of being killed. Dreams might mean something, or they might be nonsense with no meaning whatsoever. Of the dreams that have meaning, they might be related to interpersonal conflicts, sexual motivations, social concerns, a fear of embarrassment or to help solve problems in our lives.

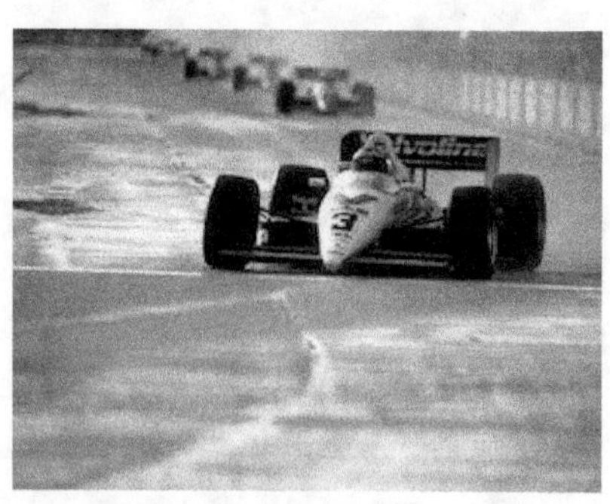

When I was a kid, I had a recurring dream that persisted for a few months. I was around 8 years old and riding in the back seat of my parent's car, a big metal monster of a vehicle that we had in the '60s. I was looking out the side window while we drove past the Lockheed Airport, a small private airport that eventually grew to become Hollywood-Burbank International Airport. The runway back then began and/or ended right at the boulevard and, as we passed, I could see a small private plane dropping straight down toward the runway. My dad punched the gas and we sped away from the crash, but I heard the impact in the distance. That's when I would wake up.

Did that dream tell me to be cautious? Was it a premonition of someone I know or myself being in a plane crash? Was my dad a hero? It could have meant something, but I never did connect it to any event. I have always felt uneasy flying in a small plane, but whether that was a result of my dream or just my discomfort with altitude is something I'll probably never figure out.

I think it might be a good thing that most dreams are not remembered. Over the years, how would we differentiate between memories and past dreams? Just think of déjà vu on steroids.

Most experts agree that dreams during REM sleep have health benefits and many studies have shown that lack of dreaming, like when subjects are awakened whenever REM sleep begins, leads to higher anxiety, stress and depression.

My dreams have themes and patterns of their own. I've noticed that often I am taken through a maze of buildings, rooms and landscapes only to find that I need to retrace my steps back. When I was young, they sort of walked me through all the bases in sexual encounters, well before I needed to know them. I used to have dreams in which I was frozen in place after seeing a rattlesnake or other danger. Many of my dreams are epic, taking hours and involving complicated storylines or scenery. Over time I tend to better remember dreams with reccurring themes like these.

Vivid dreams are those in which you are aware that you are dreaming while events unfold, often as a voyeur, a participant or both. Sometimes I become aware of my dream as I am waking up, but I typically don't fully experience vivid dreams. Sounds like it's my loss.

There are those who attach spiritual or psychological meaning to all dreams, but to me they are just the brain exercising its synapses and occasionally figuring out how to react to a problem at hand. Either way, one is almost always happier when they experience dreams than those who don't.

==================

My closing thought on this topic is captured nicely in a quote by Leonardo da Vinci, who pondered, "*Why does the eye see a thing more clearly in dreams than the imagination when awake?*"

38. Roadside Attractions

One sunny afternoon in the flat plains of Central Kansas, we came across a field with hundreds of kinetic and other metal sculptures. I had heard that there were unusual roadside attractions in the Midwest, but this was the first time I was taken aback by one. Mullinville, Kansas, is a small town on U.S. Highway 400 and its claim to fame are these "totems," as their creator, a reportedly ill-tempered M.T. Liggett, calls them. They are made from junked farm machinery, car parts, road signs or railroad equipment.

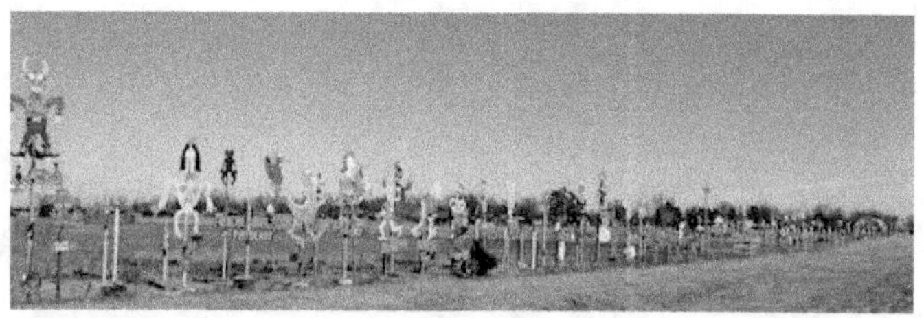

From the giant dinosaurs in Cabazon, Calif., to "Carhenge" in Alliance, Neb., to the massive "Geese in Flight" metal sculptures in North Dakota, surprises around the bend will usually delight, if not impress. There's a giant elephant in New Jersey, the world's largest thermometer in the California desert, and mammoth statues of Paul Bunyan and Babe, the Blue Ox, throughout North America. Bring your own spray paint and help decorate the upended relics at Cadillac Ranch in Amarillo, Texas.

There are literally hundreds of these attractions scattered all over America, many on out-of-the-way back roads and are the hope of each county or town near their location. What makes them special is the quirky or humorous nature of the creations, the more unexpected the better. For example, the World's Largest Ball of Yarn doesn't really cut it any longer, but New York State's "World's Largest Garden Gnome" will definitely have you cracking a smile. Beneath an overpass in Seattle, there is a cement statue, the Fremont Troll, so large that a full-size VW bug fits in its clutched hand.

There also seem to me popular themes to these attractions. Treat yourself to a visit to the UFO Welcome Center in Bowman, S.C., or to the Little A'le'inn, a roadside café and motel on the Extraterrestrial Highway in Nevada. Huge dinosaurs can be found in nearly every state, as can the "World's Largest" almost anything. There's a Foamhenge in Virginia, a replica of Stonehenge in Washington State, the aforementioned Cadillac Ranch and Carhenge, and other "Henges" of various types across the country. There are also umpteen metal horse, elk and buffalo statues on the plains and rolling hills of the Midwest and the deserts of Texas, Oklahoma and Arizona, some with Native Americans in chase.

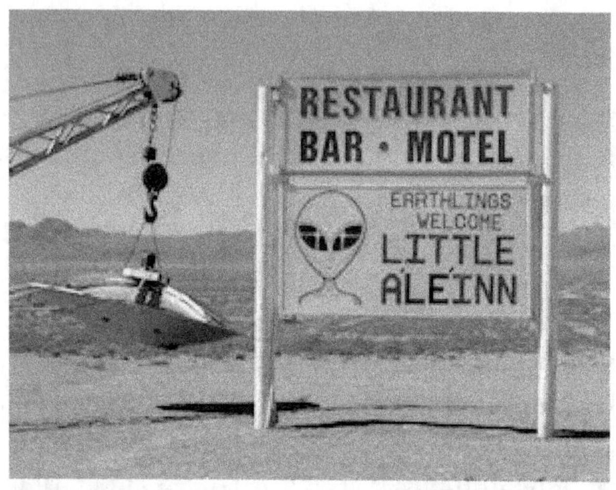

We've seen bowling ball gardens, hot-dog-shaped cafes, coffeepot or teapot gas stations, giant rocks in a myriad of shapes, and a "city" of round rocks. Ghost towns seem to be everywhere, as are an abundance of outdoor museums of farm and ranch equipment, and strange man-made structures like Bishop's Castle in Colorado. Many have expressed fascination with the over-painted Salvation Mountain in Slab City, Calif., or the Unclaimed Baggage Center in Alabama.

All told, we wouldn't enjoy life on the road as much without at least some of these respites from dreary highway travel, helping make the road less traveled much more fun.

==================

Interestingly, my closing quote typifies why interesting roadside attractions are so often missed by tourists. It was attributed to Gilbert K. Chesterton, an English writer who lived during the turn of the 20th century. He wrote, appropriately, *"The traveler sees what he sees, the tourist sees what he has come to see."*

39. Redecoration

Decorating and redecorating has been a passion of mine for decades. One of the most exciting things about moving into a new house (or new to us) is the prospect of a clean slate and letting my creative juices flow. We've lived in almost a dozen apartments, townhouses and houses since we've been together, and each one needed décor.

It's not just the end result that is satisfying, it's also the process leading up to it. I've never had formal training in home décor or interior design. It's something that seems to come naturally to me, somewhat like my photography.

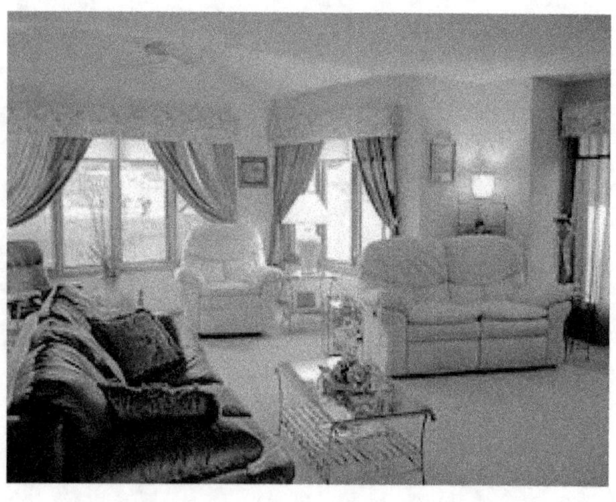

Moving into our fifth wheel full-time was a real adventure in home décor, having to juggle space and comfort and create a living space. That's quite different from using an RV for weekends. Unlike a house, remodeling an RV can be exceedingly difficult, with extra-small spaces exaggerating the features and colors. Non-standard construction and materials can make any project seem daunting or impossible.

Some see redecorating as a personal project to design and implement, some as a relief from a boring or stale existence. There are those who see it as a tedious task that might be slightly more than a necessity. Others see decorating as a totally creative endeavor. No matter the purpose, beautiful outcomes can be exceedingly rewarding. It is well-known that functioning in beautiful spaces can boost our mood and reduce stress, so improving your atmosphere will likely improve your morale.

Similar to the "new car smell" when you first bring home a new auto, redecorating can give a room or house a new look, often refreshing a worn, dingy space you had more than gotten used to. That new look can also be a springboard for inspiration in all your creative ventures. If a room is decorated in an interesting way, you are more likely to spend hours in it, comfortably examining all of its features and appreciating the eye of the decorator. It might feel like you have modernized as well, as dated decor can often become boring and "so yesterday." Remodeling can also make extra room or a construct a more exciting use for a space. Change can be good, but enhancing the use of a room can be priceless.

It doesn't take an expensive construction project either — even repainting can significantly affect the look of the space. Anyone who has seen their home space become cluttered will appreciate a cleaning out and refurbishing of the space. Purging can be a difficult but emotionally rewarding task.

Last but not least, a competent redecoration of your home will increase its value, both monetarily and in desirability. Whether you work on the project yourself, hire professionals or help an experienced crew, the result is sure to benefit you and your life in many ways.

==================

To complete this discussion, I'll quote American businessman Gary Hamel, who said, "*As human beings, we are the only organisms that create for the sheer stupid pleasure of doing so. Whether it's laying out a garden, composing a new tune on the piano, writing a bit of poetry, manipulating a digital photo, redecorating a room, or inventing a new chili recipe - we are happiest when we are creating.*"

40. Donuts

I know, I know, I already used the topic of "Chocolate" in this series. Since donuts come in more types and flavors than chocolate, and, after all, they are their own food group, donuts are the bomb and deserve their own reason for happiness.

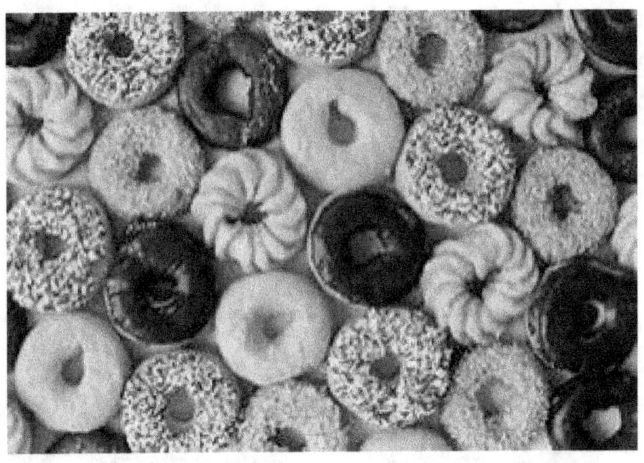

My earliest recollection of fresh-baked donuts came when I was around 8 or 9 years old in Southern California. Back then there was a bread company, Weber, that delivered bread and pastries on routes throughout the region. Later, Helm's Bakery would continue the service. Like the ice cream man and more accessible than Santa Claus, the bread truck was something all the kids in the neighborhood eagerly awaited. We saved our allowance for every Saturday during the school year and every day in the summer.

Once seen, we would race inside to grab our change and gather in one front yard or another, waving our arms until he stopped. Some mothers would come out and buy a few loaves of fresh bread and then it was our turn. He would pull out the four-foot-wide drawer holding the sweet goods in the back of the truck and the smell of fresh baked goods would ignite a frenzy. For a dime we could buy what seemed like a giant glazed donut, still warm and glaze dripping when he handed it to us in a wax paper liner. Life was good.

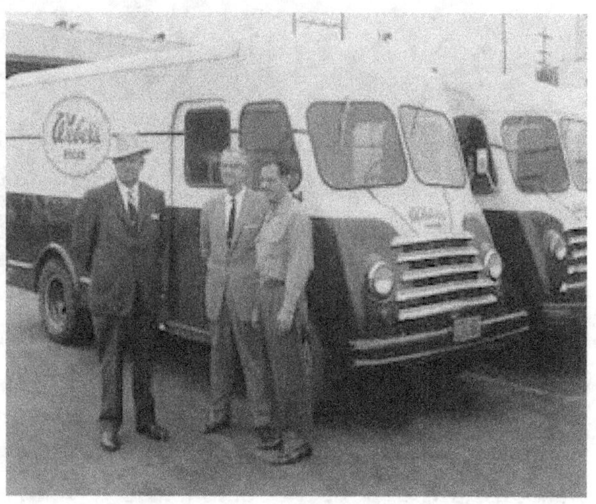

Supermarkets eventually put food delivery services, like bread and milk, out of business, and, for a long time, fresh donuts (or the quaint "doughnuts") were only really available if you fried them yourselves. Whether you are making cake or yeast (rising) donuts, what sets them apart from other pastries is that you deep fry them instead of baking. For decades the best dessert-moms made donuts with a variety of toppings. I remember helping my mother by taking a small paper sack, dumping in either powdered sugar or a mix of white sugar and cinnamon, tossing in one sizzling donut at a time and shaking the sack, now hot from the donut's frying grease, and placing each on a plate, one after another. Heaven.

Donut shops and their mass production methods didn't measure up to the bread trucks, grocery store bakeries or mom's kitchen, but were still a desirable option. Over the years, regional and national chains got better through competition and innovation, and in the past 10 years a renaissance of sorts in donut shops has raised the quality to new heights. From L.A.'s famous drive-through Randy's Donuts (or the Donut Hole in our town), through Winchell's and Dunkin' Donuts, to the Canadian and Northeastern Tim Hortons, to the ever-popular Krispy Kreme and Daylight Donuts, and ending up with the current chains of Voodoo Donuts and Astro Donuts and Chicken, the number of extremely good donut locations are still on the rise, pun intended.

In traveling around America, we can say with confidence that Texas is the donut capital of the U.S. Almost any town there with a post office and a gas station has at least one mom-and-pop donut shop, and most have several. Like pizza in Chicago or wings in Buffalo, if you don't make great donuts in Texas, you won't stay in business. The only drawback is that you must watch your intake or your weight will definitely suffer.

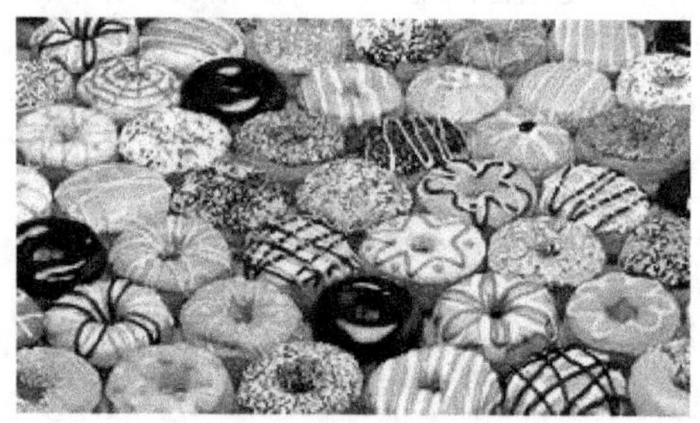

Everyone has one or more favorite types of donut. Mine are chocolate-iced glazed and chocolate bars. Nadyne favors white-frosted vanilla cake donuts with sprinkles and regular glazed. You may like your raised donuts glazed, crème-filled, custard-filled or fruit-filled. You might crave any number of types of cake donuts, French crullers (or "truck tires"), fruit fritters, long Johns, éclairs, old-fashioned, and let's not forget about twists. On top of all of these, you can mix and match recipes, fillings, frostings and toppings.

Regardless of your preference, most people like most donuts, and sometimes any old genre will do. It's one of the only food groups that allows that kind of flexibility. Okay, I know it's not a real food group, but I rather enjoy my fantasy.

==================

It seems appropriate to finish this topic with a quote from American pastry chef, food writer and YouTube personality, Claire Saffitz, who said, "*The first time I ever deep-fried something, I was terrified. I was making yeasted jelly donuts, and I was so nervous that I fried them, unblinking, with a pounding heart and sweaty palms.*"

41. Wine

It's only fair, after touting the benefits of craft beer, that I include wine as a reason for happiness. After all, I've been drinking wine for over 30 years and still enjoy stopping at wineries for tasting.

Wine has been produced for thousands of years. According to Wikipedia, the earliest evidence of wine is from ancient Georgia (6000 BC), Persia (5000 BC), and Italy (4000 BC). New World wine has some connection to alcoholic beverages made by the indigenous peoples of the Americas, but is mainly connected to the later Viking area of Vinland and Spanish traditions in New Spain. We can thank Europeans for developing wine and the industry to what it is today, but it is produced in most countries in the world.

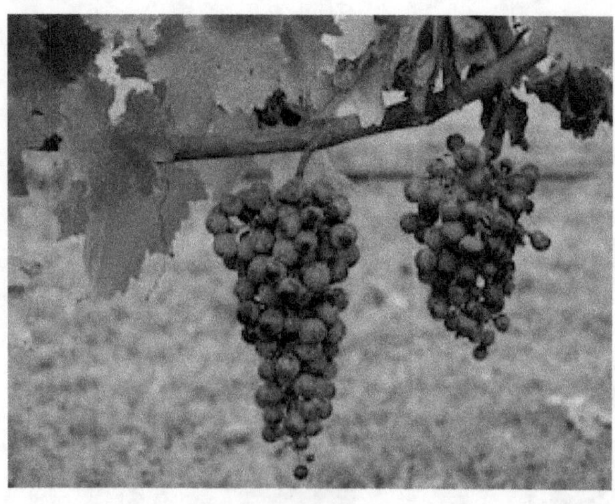

Like the world, the United States has also had a bit of a wine producing explosion, with states that don't grow grapes well simply importing from those that do. I was fortunate to live in the midst of the Washington State wine country when I first started to imbibe. Back in the '80s there were almost 100 wineries in the Yakima Valley Wine Country, and let's just say my home was Wine-Country-adjacent. I found most winery owners more than pleased to talk to visitors and many insisted on giving personal tours of their facilities.

Similar to most wine novices, I started drinking sweet wines, such as Rieslings, Gewürztraminers and blushes. Over time, my taste changed and these began to taste as sweet as Kool-Aid. I was ready to go dry. Two years later, I was heavily into Chardonnay, Sauvignon Blanc and Pinot Grigio for whites and started delving into some red wines. Soon I was drinking Merlot, Cabernet Sauvignon, Pinot Noir and Zinfandel. I can no longer drink anything remotely sweet. And blends! Those glorious red blends from Spain and Italy are wine nirvana.

What makes wine different from hard alcohol is the process and alcohol content. Both use fermentation to convert sugar or starch to alcohol, but hard spirits like vodka, whiskey and rum add a distillery process. Wine typically has a 9-16 percent alcohol content, while hard spirits are normally 28-

60 percent, depending on the product. Compare that to beer at 3-9 percent ABV (alcohol by volume), and it is easy to see that beer and wine allow more beverage to be enjoyed before inebriation (if you can say "inebriation" aloud without stumbling over it, you probably aren't experiencing it).

The medical and health benefits of drinking wine are numerous. Studies have shown that compounds found in red wine tannins help promote cardiovascular health, and occupants of those regions of the world in which wine is part of the normal diet tend to live longer. Researchers in Spain found that adults who drank two to seven glasses of wine per week were less likely to be diagnosed with depression. Modest wine consumption, meaning one glass a day, may decrease the prevalence of Non-Alcoholic Fatty Liver Disease. Wine's antimicrobial effects on the skin also helps reduce bacteria on our teeth. There are many studies suggesting that the risks of various cancers are reduced by consuming red wine.

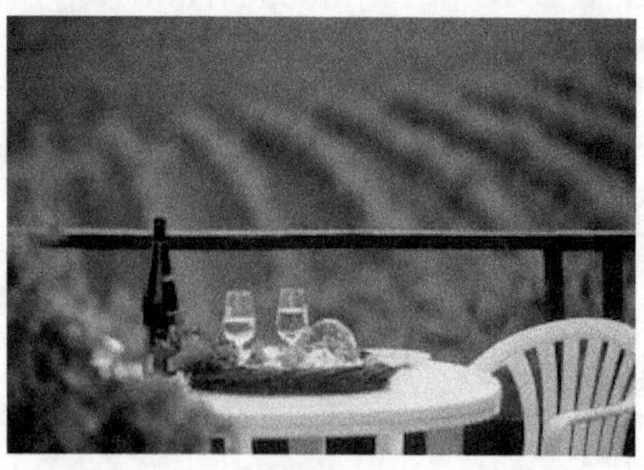

Aside from wine's health benefits, it also provides you with various social benefits. It can boost one's confidence and help overcome shyness. Being drunk is an anti-social behavior, so I am discussing wine in moderation. Similarly, drinking wine in social settings can help you connect with others and expose you to different people and places than you are used to. Wine itself can be a conversation starter and many friendships have developed over the love of wine.

What candlelit dinner is complete without wine or a celebration without champaign? Wine has been used in romance and ceremony for as long as wine has been produced. Wine and nature go hand-in-hand, just as wine and travel enhance each other.

Another great thing about wine is its effect on the taste of food. There is a reason there are suggested wine pairings for most of the meals you enjoy. Red wine tends to cleanse the palate between bites of beef or pasta, while tones of white wines can enhance the flavor of poultry and pork dishes. For every food offering, a perfect wine variety can be found to maximize the enjoyment of its consumption.

The advent of craft beer has crept into what was once wine's sole environment, but it is not a total social replacement. There are times I want beer, for example, in long nights of sports viewing or playing, since the alcohol content can dictate the duration of the entertainment. But wine is still my go-to drink for feast and cheer. I rarely drink hard alcohol, which usually makes for short nights, and sipping my wine is much more pleasurable than downing shots.

All told, wine is a luxury in which everyone can indulge, and with the wide range of flavors and sweetness, there is a wine for almost everybody and every occasion.

==================

To complete the discussion, I'll include the shortest quote I've used thus far. Nineteenth-century Scottish author Robert Louis Stevenson once said, "*Wine is bottled poetry.*" I just can't argue the point.

42. Camping and Glamping

My parents never took me camping, not that Los Angeles has ever been a camper's nirvana. They did, though, support my joining the local Boy Scouts troop, the leaders of which took the members camping a few times a year. We visited the Angeles and San Bernardino National Forests, the Mojave Desert and other areas around Southern California. I vividly remember hiking to one of the peaks in the San Gabriel Mountains and shivering in the cold because I had failed to anticipate and pack for 30-degree temps at nearly 8,000 feet.

Even so, I loved camping and enjoyed it as often as I could over the years. When my oldest daughter was less than a year old, we camped in the Yosemite National Forest, and she was no worse for wear from the experience. I think all of my kids enjoyed the experiences we had after moving to Washington State. Camping and fishing were two of our primary activities every summer.

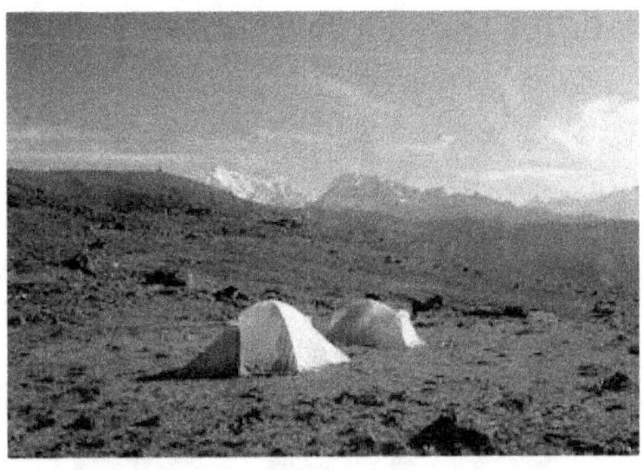

The kids grew up and I moved to Western New York, and camping was less available, so for years it was a forgotten habit. It wasn't until my wife and I moved to Las Vegas and realized we both had the itch to travel and see America that my vagabond nature returned. However, this time it would be glamping, not just camping. "Glamping," or "glamor camping," is the term some people give to camping in RVs rather than tents. As you get older, tent-camping becomes much less desirable.

Campouts are not just for families any more -- we actually camp full-time. One of the popular aspects of camping is the huge variety of types and styles available to the average person. Even tents have improved to the point where they may not even be recognizable as such. Canvas cabins are as spacious as wooden ones. Hard-side pull-trailers and traditional tent trailers have been combined into "hybrid" camping trailers. Fifth wheel trailers can range from small 20-foot rigs to huge 45-foot toy haulers and you can utilize from one to five or more slide-outs for even more space. Several have side and/or rear raised decks.

Then there are the myriad of types of motorhomes, from a regular van conversion, rated a class B, to a larger and more sophisticated class B+, to the traditional class C motorhome on a larger chassis and truck cab with the usual overhang for a bed or storage, to a bus style class A. The lines between the styles and classes are being blurred more each season. Glamping just doesn't get any better, or more expensive.

No discussion about styles of camping would be complete without defining the types of camping. It is estimated that there are over 15,000 RV resorts, parks and campgrounds in the U.S., and they range from rustic forest or state campgrounds without or with limited hookups, to more traditional parks with or without full hookups, to neighborhoods of park model or manufactured homes that allow RVs, full-service RV resorts with amenities that never end. If you want to rough it, you can boondock or dry camp, which is basically picking a spot in a forest or meadow, on the plains or in the desert, and making camp without any services or amenities except what you brought for yourself. Fortunately, most RVs are completely self-contained, sporting water and waste tanks and a generator or solar system for power, so a week or less is totally possible to enjoy in this manner.

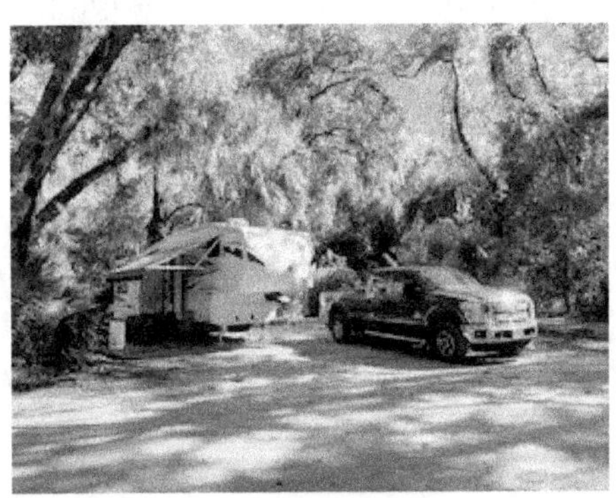

Communing with nature is never better than when you experience it while camping. Usually, the location you choose will provide plenty of fresh air, and often hiking or biking is readily available relatively close by. So, the health benefits are all around you, including a reduction of stress and a happier mood. That feeling of glee you get when you take your first breath of air in a campground isn't all in your mind -- it's due to a release of serotonin from breathing in the extra oxygen produced by trees and in the forest. When you are out in direct sunlight, you're receiving an abundance of vitamin D, which allows your body to better absorb calcium and phosphorous. Even mild activity usually equates to a good night's sleep, and the natural surroundings may allow or even suggest some soothing meditation.

RVers and other campers are ordinarily a social bunch, so it is easy to make new and long-lasting friendships. This is true whether you camp over a weekend, over a season or full-time. Not only did we make lifelong friends while camping in Colorado, but developed a surprising number of friends and acquaintances we met after hitting the road a few short years ago.

There are many ways that camping or glamping can provide happiness in your life. It did that for us in such abundance that it is now our daily way of life.

=================

I'll close the subject with a quote from a British politician, Margaret Beckett, who experienced glamping: "*Some people think that going on a caravan holiday is a slightly more upscale version of camping. Let me assure you, it is much better than that. You know that you will have your creature comforts wherever you are. I never have to pack light, and I can put the kettle on in any location.*"

43. Television

Mine was the first generation that has been entirely entertained at home by television shows, albeit they were black-and-white when I was a kid. Before that, perhaps unbelievably so, families would pull up chairs to the living room radio and listen to their favorite episodes of *Ozzie and Harriet*, *Abbott and Costello*, *Burns and Allen*, *Jack Benny*, *Life of Riley*, *The Lone Ranger*, or one of hundreds broadcast in the '40s and '50s. Many of those were the first television series as well, since they already had an audience and sponsors. Soon, though, the vision part of television added a new dimension to entertainment and shows began rolling out for that medium.

I wasn't planning on making this a history lesson, but I thought I was reminisce for a moment. I vividly remember kid shows growing up, like *Rin Tin Tin*, *Roy Rogers*, *Flipper*, the aforementioned *Lone Ranger*, *Superman*, *Sky King*, *The Rifleman*, *Kukla Fran and Ollie*, *Sherri Lewis*, and a myriad of cartoons (like *Johnny Quest*, *Bugs Bunny*, *Huckleberry Hound* and *Mighty Mouse*). As I got older, on came *Star Trek*, *Batman*, *I Dream of Jeanie*, *Lost in Space*, *Andy Griffith*, *Bewitched*, *Hogan's Heroes*, *Gilligan's Island*, *I Spy* and so many more. There were many genres created for broadcast, with westerns, sci-fi, variety, police and medical dramas, horror, morning and daytime, news, game shows, sports and sitcoms, short for "situation comedies."

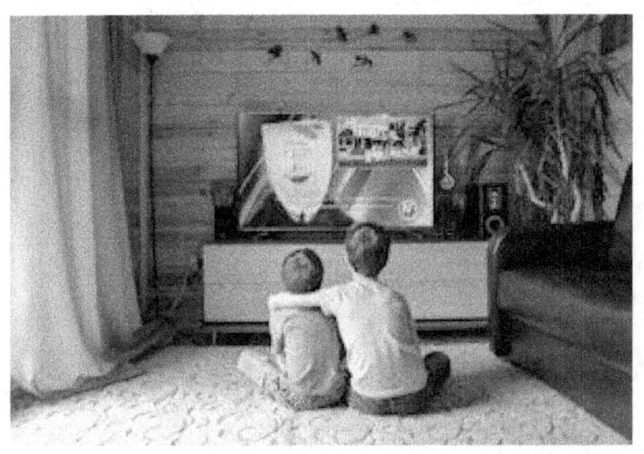

On the road full-time, we have an even better appreciation for a good TV series. Nighttime in the wilderness or in a remote campground has limited entertainment opportunities. There are only so many times you want to sit around a campfire, and we're often too removed from any nightlife for it to be an option. With the advent of the mobile satellite dish and streaming services, we have just about all the TV we want. We have a nightly ritual of streaming old series, like *How I Met Your Mother*, *Frasier*, and *In Plain Sight*, one episode per evening for two or three shows. It took several months to complete all 13 seasons of *Frasier*, one show per night.

Besides its entertainment value, television can be educational and cultural, providing insights into people and places you have never experienced. We still get our national and local news via the TV. Being part of a fanbase can be fun and give you something to talk about to friends, family and new acquaintances. There is no better way to be a sports fan than watching your favorite team on the tube, and, better yet, inviting all your friends and family over to share the experience. TV shows can also help you feel less lonely, allowing you to involve yourself in the characters' relationships. Watching DIY, cooking and outdoors shows can inspire you to try new things or pick up a new hobby.

Watching TV is also an excellent bonding opportunity for you and your life partner or close friend. It can be a significant shared experience or just a nice enjoyable time, either being beneficial to your relationship. If you sit together while watching, you can have intimate moments and touch, and even with a scary scene, provide valuable physical and emotional support.

You have probably heard the old adage, "Laughter is the best medicine." Television comedies can improve your health and mental state in this way and studies have found that people feel more energetic after watching nature shows on TV.

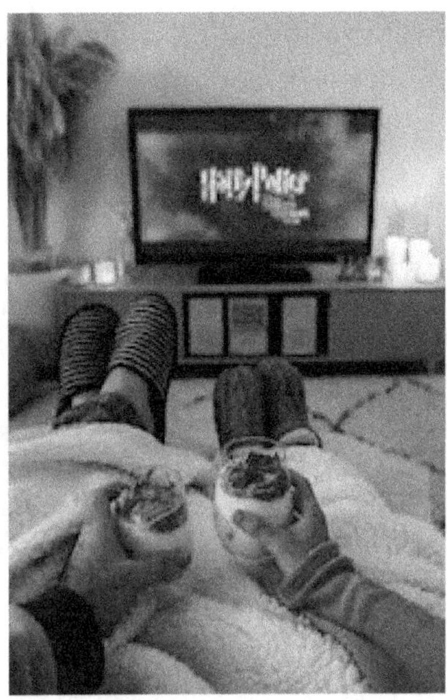

It has been reported that watching TV can reduce stress and your cortisol levels, high levels of which can cause weight gain, higher bad cholesterol and depression.

Last, it is among the least expensive forms of entertainment, as long as you monitor all of your monthly subscribed service fees. You can easily have more television than you can watch for less than $100 per month.

Whether you are a home body, an avid camper or a full-time RVer, television is a huge safety net against boredom and stagnation of your imagination, and can provide a wonderful source of happiness. Just remember, when it stops being enjoyable, there is an on-off switch.

=================

The final word in the subject comes from American actor Melissa Rauch, who said, *"TV was my life, growing up. I ran home from school to watch television, and even did my homework with the TV on - my mom had a rule that as long as my grades didn't fall, I was allowed to. So it was my dream to work in television."*

44. Mountains

Nadyne and I grew up near mountains, she in Tucson, Ariz., and me in the Los Angeles Basin in Southern California. We share a love of mountain views and their majesty. But, like the song lyrics go, "Don't it always seem to go that you don't know what you've got 'til it's gone?" We moved to Kansas, where the nearest mountains were almost 300 miles away. In fact, we used to joke that from the 12th floor in the Wichita City Hall you could see all the way to the Gulf of Mexico. Sorry, Flat-Earthers, the curvature of the earth kept this from being true.

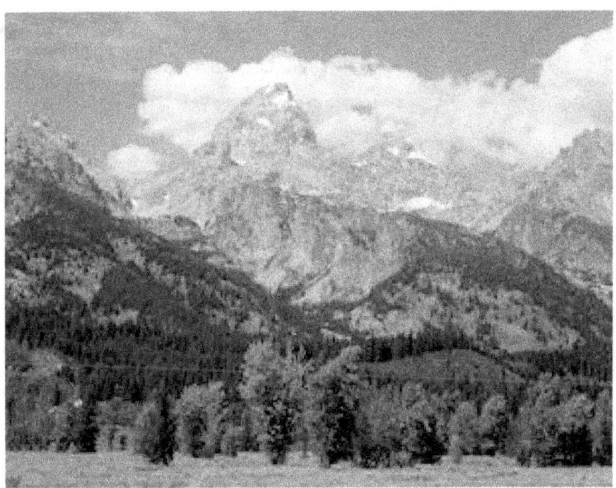

We experienced an interesting phenomenon in Wichita that extended to many flat plains locations: claustrophobia. How can being in a wide-open space cause such a feeling? I finally figured out that it has to do with a finite horizon. Walk or drive anywhere with mountains and the sight of the range gives you an internal sense of the size of the space you are in. Take away the mountains and either you have a non-distinct view of the infinite horizon or the horizon becomes the building rooflines, treetops or the top edges of tall hedges. That loss of a distinct space can be unnerving to those of us who grew up around mountains, and it didn't seem to affect native Kansans at all.

Believe it or not, there are health benefits to visiting a mountain range. There are several reports that spending almost any time in the mountains can trigger weight loss and high altitude is known to decrease your appetite and make you feel more full. People who live in or spend considerable time at higher altitudes, which would include cities like Denver, Colo., and Santa Fe, N.M., are less likely to die from a heart attack and have lower risk of cardiovascular disease. The fresh air you breathe in the mountains, free of toxic gasses and air pollution, gives your lungs a chance to breathe in a better mix of oxygen. Pine scents also tend to decrease hostility, depression and stress. Mountain trails also provide some of the best exercise available and the opportunity for bonding with friends, family and that special someone.

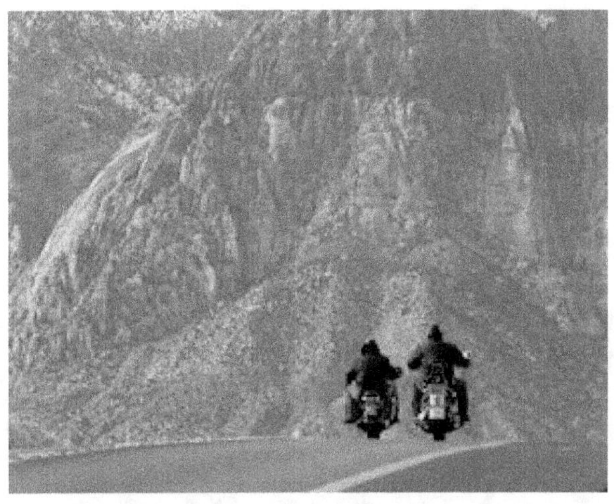

You can extend all the benefits I embraced with trees to the mountains as well, since more trees inhabit mountainous regions than all other geographical zones combined. Speaking of geography, and therefore geology, there are three major ways mountains form, all as a byproduct of plate tectonics. Volcanic activities occur when one tectonic plate is pushed beneath another, causing magma to be forced to the surface. The "Ring of Fire" was created in this manner, as have the series of dormant volcanoes in the Cascades, site of Mount St. Helens. During tectonic plate collisions, when two plates plow into each other, one plate is forced upwards, creating ranges such as the Appalachians, Himalayas and Mount Everest. The least-known is rifting, when rocks on one side of a fault lift relative to the opposite side, such as with the Black Forest in Germany. I don't want to make this a geology course, but as we tour America, it is interesting to see how the different mountain ranges were created and how they have changed over geologic time.

The "purple mountains majesty," though, is why we love to visit the mountains, with photos not exactly doing them justice, and with views sometimes so amazing as to render us awestruck in silence.

==================

I'll complete this discussion with a quote from a famous 19th-century novelist, Nathaniel Hawthorne, who wrote, *"Mountains are earth's undecaying monuments."*

45. Ghost Towns

One of the great adventures you can take, especially in the West and Midwest, is to search for ghost towns. You might define a ghost town as one that was abandoned by its inhabitants, usually because of a business decline.   A nearby mine may have been worked out, a large dominant company may have closed its doors or an environmental or weather-related disaster may have chased residents away. When we come across one, it is both sad and fascinating.

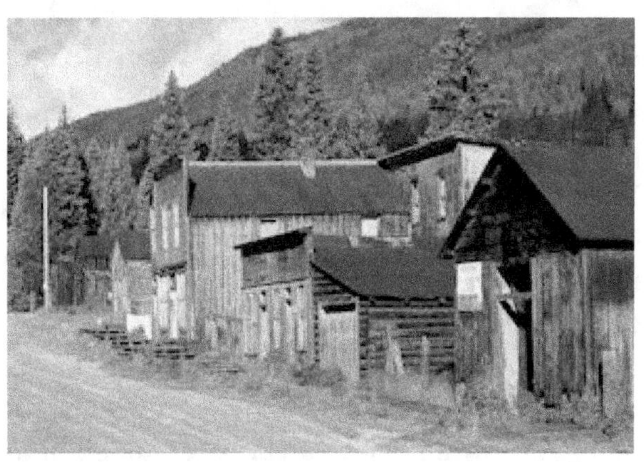

Goldfield, Nev., was one of the first ghost towns I've ever visited, though, to be fair, there are still a bit over 200 residents listed in its official population. That is a far stretch from its heyday as the largest city in Nevada, when the population was around 20,000 in about 1904 to 1906. During that time another bit of history was made there, when Wyatt and Virgil Earp arrived. Virgil was hired as a Goldfield deputy sheriff in January 1905, but in October he died of pneumonia after six months of illness. Wyatt Earp left Goldfield shortly afterward. By 1910, the population was down below 5,000 and by 1912 the largest mining company shut down operations. A fire due to a moonshine explosion destroyed most of Goldfield's wooden buildings in 1923, and the town continued to decline until it became what we see today.

To be able to read about that kind of detail about a town's history is unusual, mostly available because of the tourist draw. Most ghost towns have limited documentation, but sometimes that makes the find even more interesting, our imaginations placed in high gear to fill in the blanks. Some, like Tombstone in Southern Arizona, Calico in Southern California and St. Elmo in Central Colorado, have renovated or reconstructed many of its buildings in order to draw tourists. Others, such as Gila City and Fortuna, both outside of Yuma, Ariz., are barren or badly neglected. More and more, however, are being renovated due to an apparent need of new attractions for tourists.

I remember seeing several rows of abandoned two-story houses and other buildings when we were on our way to check out the quaint town of Red Cliff, Colo. We could see the remnants of a mining operation and assumed it was a closed company town. A little research told us that it was indeed an abandoned mining town called Gilman that had operated from 1886 until the mine closed in 1984 by the Environmental Protection Agency, as well as its unprofitability. Apparently, in mining large quantities of lead and zinc, the mine contaminated the groundwater with toxic chemicals. You can't get close to the buildings, but with a telephoto lens or binoculars you can see household items and furniture still sitting inside.

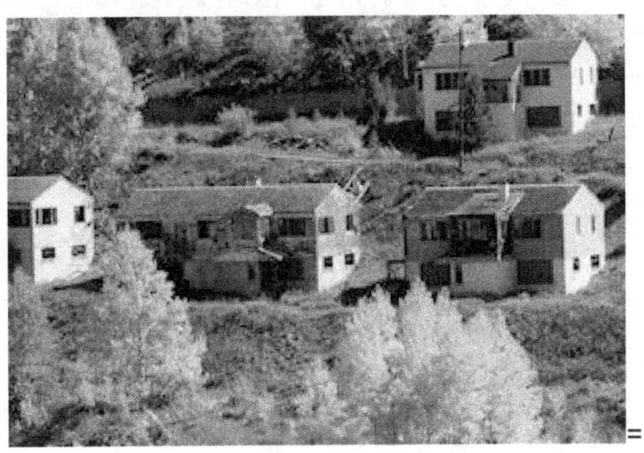

Another cultural phenomenon has created a new tourist boom — haunted towns that put the "ghost" in ghost towns. One of the most popular is Bodie, Calif. As with most mining towns in the 19th century, the business of sin took advantage of the gold being pulled from the mines. All of that crime, greed and lust took its toll and, when the town was abandoned, stories remained of paranormal experiences, especially in the home of a man named

Jim Cain. An Asian servant took her own life there after being fired and ever since there have been numerous reports of the sound of music from a particular bedroom, the face of a woman eerily appearing at a second-story window, individuals feeling as if they are being held down, and others. Bodie was also reportedly cursed as well. I'm not into paranormal experiences, but if you are, ghost towns can be a gold mine, pun intended.

Like geocaching, locating and exploring ghost towns are extremely enjoyable activities, getting you outdoors and walking or hiking about the area. There is much information about which ghost towns are in any particular region or state, often including directions and/or GPS coordinates. When we have taken on such an outing, there is a real possibility of not finding some of the towns, since roads leading to them have often been abandoned or torn up, and that there may well be nothing to find. But, that's half the fun, right?

==================

To complete this topic, I'll end with a quote from American actor Hong Chau, who said, *"I'm really into ghost towns. I've driven cross-country the past few summers, and I would stop at some ghost towns along the way. They're like a microcosm of America as a whole."*

46. Good Health

When you have your health, you have everything. In my opinion, truer words were never spoken. Quality of life is almost as important as life itself. Fortunately for the Baby Boomer and subsequent generations, longer lifespans also include better medicine, better fitness, no smoking and less age-related maladies. Once cancer is licked, the human lifespan will take another large step.

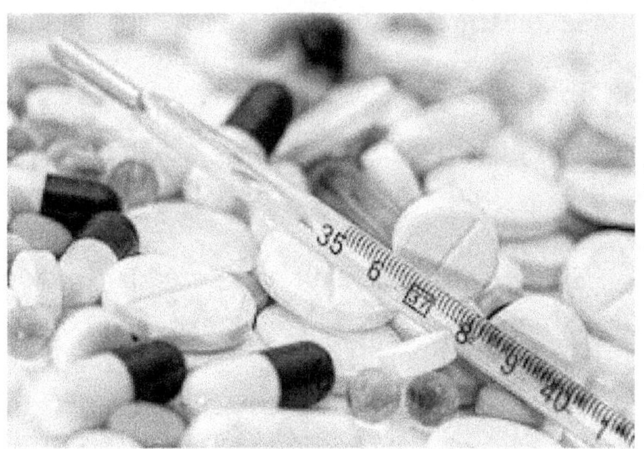

When I was 10 and my grandparents were in their 60s, they looked like 85-year-olds today. I have seen family photos of them, so I can assure you that it wasn't just my view of them as a youngster. They looked *old*. Now in my 60s myself, I can appreciate how lucky I am. When they say that

65 is the new 45, there is some truth to the statement.

When you think of all the health risks someone born at the turn of the 20th century had to endure, you have to wonder how they survived to have a family at all. Penicillin wasn't discovered until 1928. The existence of vitamins was only suggested in 1906. Insulin wasn't used to treat diabetes until 1922, just before the first vaccines were developed for diphtheria, whooping cough, tuberculosis, and tetanus. The first flu vaccine wasn't given until 1945. Pacemakers were invented in 1952 and the polio vaccine was developed in 1955. You can see that medicine has been a great boon to the human race over the decades. Just think of life without all of these wonder drugs and miracle treatments.

Good health has been hampered by smoking more than any other human activity, and death from tobacco use is the leading preventable cause of death in the U.S., still causing about one in five deaths each year, according to the CDC. But death isn't the only detrimental outcome from smoking. My mom contracted emphysema from smoking all her life and was on oxygen for her last 10 years. She spent the last half-dozen years in and out of hospitals.

But, let's focus on the positive. Each year, about 1.3 million smokers quit, and, since 1965, more than

40 percent of all adults who have ever smoked have quit. Recent miracle cures and treatments for cancer, heart disease and other ailments abound, and science has provided stem cell treatments, DNA analysis, gene therapy, artificial organs and this past year proved the value of lightning speed vaccine development. There are even more miracles on the horizon, like 3D printing of organs and other body parts, diagnoses by crowd-sourcing or via mobile intelligence, the use of bio-hackers, which will be ultra-sensors in your body or clothing, antibiotic "smart bombs" for directly destroying bugs in your system, and much more.

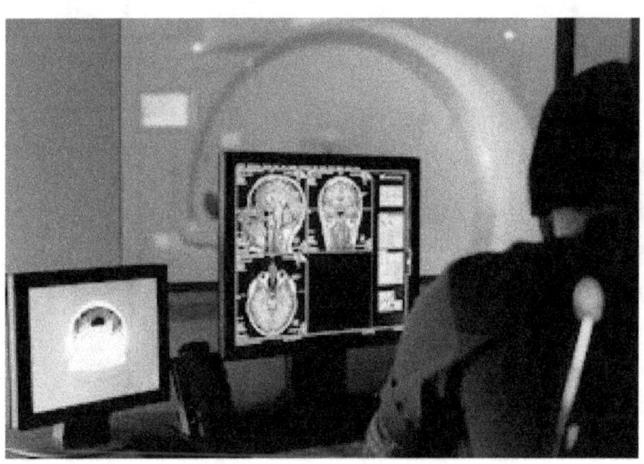

It is a good time to be a human being, and the younger generations are even more fortunate. Good health provides a happier life, with less stress and fear of contracting a serious disease and allowing you to better enjoy your hobbies and other favorite activities. A healthy person gets to spend more and better quality time with their life partners and other loved ones, and will experience less pain in their lifetime. Good health will save a lot of time and money than the alternative, with fewer medical procedures and doctor visits, and with preventive medicine being a lot less costly and stressful. You'll live longer, too, and will want to.

COVID-19 highlighted just how much we enjoy life when not faced with sickness or death in the family. There is no doubt that our quality of life is directly affected by our health and the continuous improvements in medical care.

=================

To highlight just how long health has been known to be important to one's life, here's a quote from 18th-century German philosopher Arthur Schopenhauer: *"The greatest of follies is to sacrifice health for any other kind of happiness."*

47. Books

For the younger generations, let me explain that a "book" is a bound set of paper pages with writing or printed text and/or illustrations or photos. That's a far cry from the first known attempts by people to transcribe symbols onto stone tablets, which began in about 3500 BC. A millennium later, the first known papyrus scrolls with written words were created in Egypt, with reeds and bird feathers as the probable scribing tools. A more formal writing system emerged in Europe starting in about 600 BC and the current standardized writing system slowly developed in the centuries that followed. Paper was invented in China at the turn of the 1st century AD and illustrations were added to the text starting about 400 AD. The very first printed book appeared in China in 868 AD and movable type was invented 200 years later, also in China. Movable type was first used in Europe to produce the Gutenberg Bible in 1455 and the very first book was published in America in 1639. The rest, as they say, is history. Ebooks are simply electronic versions of the same instruments but require a device with which to read them.

Books (and ebooks) can be divided into types, or genres, and all of them can be classified as fiction or non-fiction. Fiction, which consists of stories that are made-up or greatly embellished, includes many you have heard of, such as drama, horror, mystery, romance, science fiction and others. Non-fiction, or factual books, may be science, philosophy, humor, history, self-help, travel, true crime or other genres. To further complicate matters, recent trends include combining two or more genres to make new categories.

Whether you love epic adventures or are looking for some help in the kitchen, books can add a whole new dimension of pleasure to your life. They can provide mental stimulation, which can slow, or possibly even prevent, the progress of Alzheimer's and dementia. Losing yourself in a great story can reduce stress in your daily life. You can expand your knowledge by reading, as well as expand your vocabulary, helping you become better at making conversation and becoming more articulate. Both of these benefits can increase your self-esteem and improve your impact at work. Reading can also increase your empathy and improve your conversation, besides giving you some great entertainment.

Most successful authors were avid readers long before they began writing in earnest. As a teen, I loved science fiction and police dramas, so Isaac Asimov's *Foundation* and *I, Robot* series, Heinlein's *Stranger in a Strange Land* and *Time Enough for Love*, Frank Herbert's *Dune* series and *The Dosadi Experiment*, and Joseph Wambaugh's *The Onion Field* and *The New Centurions*, were all among my favorites, and I re-read each of them several times. As an adult, my attention turned more to sports fiction and non-fiction, as well as science and industry features. I am extremely pleased to have written my own retired detective series and, who knows?, maybe a sci-fi series will be next.

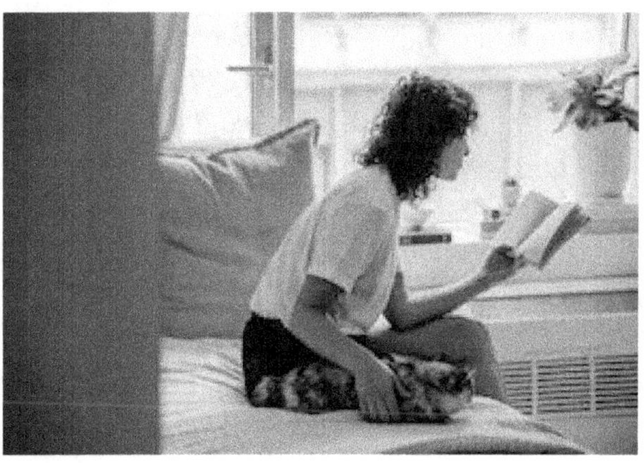

The advantage of paper books over their electronic cousins should be obvious — no device or electricity is necessary, at least in the daytime, to enjoy them. You can grab a thick Shakespeare play, a thin Harlequin romance paperback or one of the seemingly endless personal help guides, then head to the beach, the mountains, a back yard lounge chair or in front of a flickering campfire and lose yourself in ways that watching television or movies can't match. Reading forces you to imagine the scene, the setting, the characters, the voices, while letting you think about what the plot is doing, guessing what's next or whodunit. I never finished a book quickly — I kept re-reading pages or passages to get as full a comprehension as I could manage as I moved through it. But, then again, that let me enjoy them even longer.

==================

I'll end this subject with a quote from the famous scientist and naturalist, Jane Goodall, who wrote, "*When I was 10 years old, I loved - I loved books, and I used to haunt the secondhand bookshop. And I found a little book I could just afford, and I bought it, and I took it home. And I climbed up my favorite tree, and I read that book from cover to cover. And that was Tarzan of the Apes. I immediately fell in love with Tarzan.*"

48. Fishing

My dad never had time to take me fishing, but I managed to find friends to fish with. In fact, one of my best fishing buds was so into it that he opened a tackle shop and guide service. The last time he and I fished together, we had driven up the California coast and hopped on a full-day party boat in Monterey. We each caught so many we had to stop with a couple of hours to go because our arms were too sore to hold the deep-sea rods. After processing, Jack (yes, we were a pair of Jacks) had 52 pounds of luscious filleted meat and I had 37 pounds, both the tops on the boat that day.

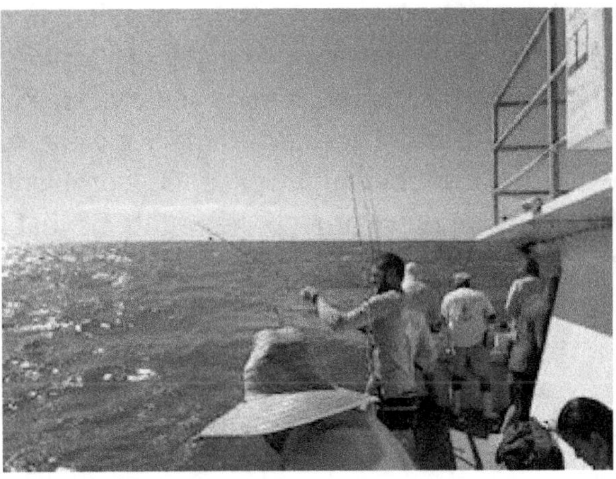

I had a few significant fishing days with other friends, too. Scott introduced me to barracuda fishing, or "backaruda," as we used to purposely mispronounce it. Barracuda feed in groups by swimming beneath large schools of anchovies and eating the small fish from the bottom, forcing the whole school up out of the water with nowhere else to go. This causes a 20- or 30-yard-wide ocean "boil" as the anchovies continually try to escape from being eaten. A fishing boat, having noticed the boil, would pull up close enough to cast across it with 12-inch-long jigs or lures. We would cast and retrieve as fast as we could, reeling in catches of the 3-4-foot-long barracuda, unhooking them in the boat and casting back out. Speed was of the essence, because the feeding frenzy could end as quickly as it erupted.

I have fished for both salt-water and fresh-water species, from shore or from a boat, guided or not, in a dozen or so states, including Alaska, Florida, California, Washington, Kansas and others. I'm looking forward to getting a Texas license as soon as we settle in at our winter space. One problem with fishing as we move around the country is that I have to purchase a non-resident license wherever I go. Florida conveniently sells annual licenses to out-of-staters, but they seem to be the exception. All-in-all, non-resident license cost keeps fishing from being a desirable activity everywhere we visit.

There are many things about angling that can make you happy, starting with the adage that a bad day of fishing is still better than a good day of working.

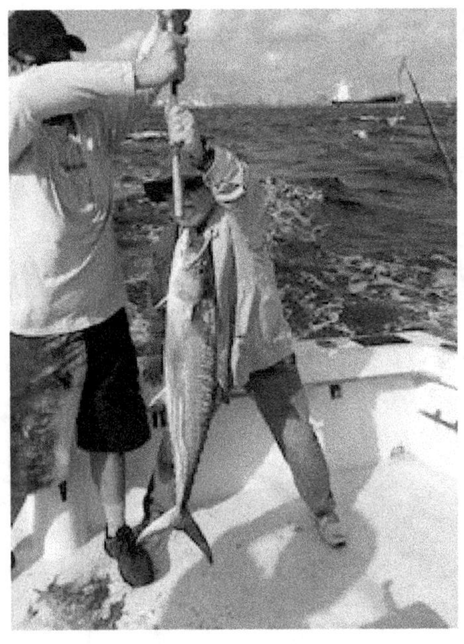

Experiencing nature and wildlife is always something I appreciate, and the entire pace of the sport is calming. It's difficult to feel stressed when you are watching your pole for a bite. Like many outdoor activities, sharing them with friends and family can help strengthen those relationships. Like camping, you can improve your self-esteem by learning to master several outdoor skills at once. Many a great fishing spot requires a long or strenuous hike (or it probably wouldn't be so great), another physical activity to improve your health. Then there's the thrill of the catch and the taste of the freshly grilled feast.

Fishing is a lifetime skill and can be enjoyed at any age. I've been fishing for over 50 years and I don't plan on stopping anytime soon.

================

There is a great quote from President Herbert Hoover that would be appropriate to share here: *"Fishing is much more than fish. It is the great occasion when we may return to the fine simplicity of our forefathers."*

49. GPS Navigation

It's 1970 and you are driving across the country to visit family several states away. Every couple of hours, you stop in at a filling station (which is what they used to call gas stations) and pull out a folded paper map and slowly unfold it on your lap. When the map exceeds the space there, you get out and open it up on the hood of the car. After several minutes of studying the map, you locate approximately where you are on the highway and decide the best route for the next couple of hours. It takes three tries and 10 minutes to fold the map, probably not the way it came, and you climb back in your car and continue the drive, hoping that you remember the turns ahead. A couple of hours later, you repeat the process, since the last thing you want is to be lost in a section of the country in which you've never been before.

Once you get to your destination city, your stop in a filling station there includes getting a local street map. Again, you unfold and study it on your hood, this time looking the street name up in the street list on the back and searching for the pertinent coordinates on the map that was listed. When you can't find it on the map, you ask the gas attendant for help and he cheerfully, or not so cheerfully, gives you directions to the address of your Aunt Martha's house, but too fast to write them down. After making three wrong turns, you miraculously find a street that had been mentioned by the attendant and you finally arrive.

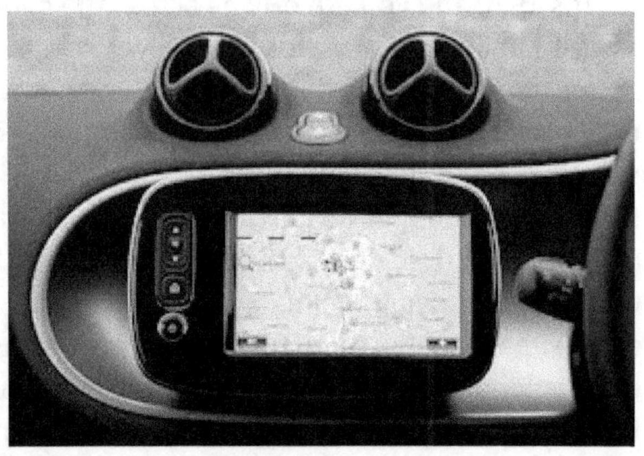

That was life before GPS navigation. I grew up working for my dad in his filling station and one of my jobs was to supply maps and directions to lost or frustrated motorists. Compare that process to our present one, in which we pull up the navigation app or GPS device on the dashboard, enter the address, wait a minute, and the first direction is read to you by a lovely disembodied voice. Yes, we have many reasons to be happy about GPS navigation.

The U.S. began the use of satellites in global positioning of submarines in the '60s, utilizing radio signals from six satellites orbiting the poles and the "Doppler effect" of shifting of signals to locate the nuclear-weapon-bearing subs in a matter of minutes. In the '70s, the U.S. Department of Defense developed a more robust navigation system using 24, then 33, satellites (NAVSTAR). Today, free GPS is available continuously to the U.S. and other governments and military, contractors of the military, corporations and the public, with accuracy predicated on the level of service.

Both geolocation and time information are utilized by cell phones, GPS devices and locater tags worldwide. In 2000, public GPS receivers had about a 16-foot accuracy range, but, in 2018, a much more accurate location service was allowed, now within about 11 inches.   Besides navigation, there are other important uses of global positioning systems, such as locating or tracking your or your family while in the field, hiking, exploring, etc. This can be especially important in an emergency, even in your vehicle. Installing a tracking device in your car will allow you to track it if it is stolen. There are even GPS tracking devices you can put on your pets' collars. Many businesses with fleets of trucks use GPS tracking to manage the trucks and their progress.

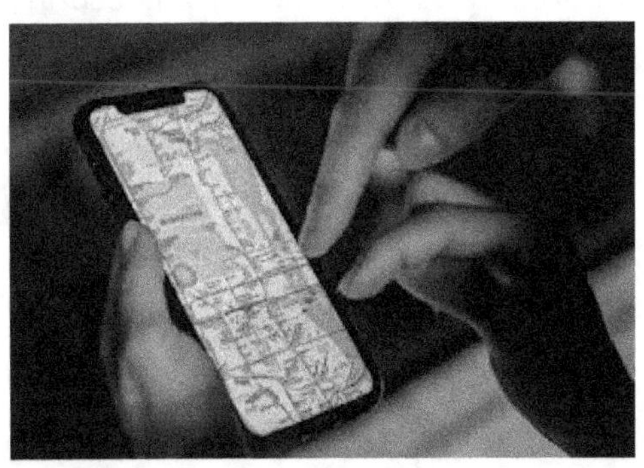

Another interesting fact about GPS navigation is that it proved Einstein's Theory of Relativity. According to phys.org, "As predicted by Einstein's theory, clocks under the force of gravity run at a slower rate than clocks viewed from a distant region experiencing weaker gravity. This means that clocks on Earth observed from orbiting satellites run at a slower rate. To have the high precision needed for GPS, this effect needs to be taken into account or there will be small differences in time that would add up quickly, calculating inaccurate positions." Thank you, Mr. Einstein. We continue to be in your debt.

==================

To complete this discussion, I'll quote American comedian Judy Gold, who said, "*I have decided now that my mother should be the GPS woman, don't you think? That would be fantastic: 'Make a left in 11 miles. Get over now - I want you to be prepared. Turn right on Elm Street, I want to see if Myrna Rosenblatt is still alive. Make your second left by the Dairy Queen. Don't go in, they're anti-Semitic.'*"

50. Bridges

Bridges can be physical structures that span and provide passage over rivers, bays, lakes, canyons, railroad tracks, roads or other barriers to travel, but can also connect two segments of music, support your cue in billiards, provide raised views from a platform on a boat or ship, or support your nose on your face. A bridge can also connect people of differing viewpoints or cultures. Here, though, I'm talking about the physical structure you can traverse on foot, by bike or in a car.

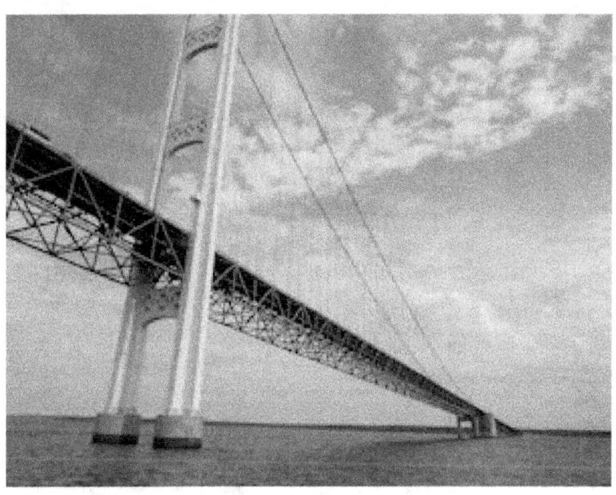

If you ever doubt how you might be taking bridges for granted, you'll be reminded when one is out on your journey. We have had to take up to five-hour detours because a bridge over a river was blocked by construction, not counting the times when the destination was simply not available by any detour at all. Just think what driving would be like without the high-tech structures that bridges have become. There was a time when the only possible passage over a river was via ferry or barge. Gorges were impassible, and some railroad tracks were blocked for hours by train traffic.

A bridge can also be a friend of the amateur or professional photographer, providing scenes of technology, history, majesty and comparable size. These views can be anything from quaint to awe-inspiring. I love shooting rustic covered bridges in Ohio and New England, but also the enormous, towering bridges that span lakes, bays and canyons. Memorable behemoths include the Golden Gate Bridge in San Francisco, Michigan's "Big Mac" over the Straits of Mackinac in the Great Lakes, the Penobscot Narrows Bridge in Maine, the New River Gorge Bridge in Virginia and the curved Chesapeake Bay Bridge in Maryland. All around the country, you'll find the picturesque, the awesome, the beautiful and the historic, if this is a photographic subject you enjoy.

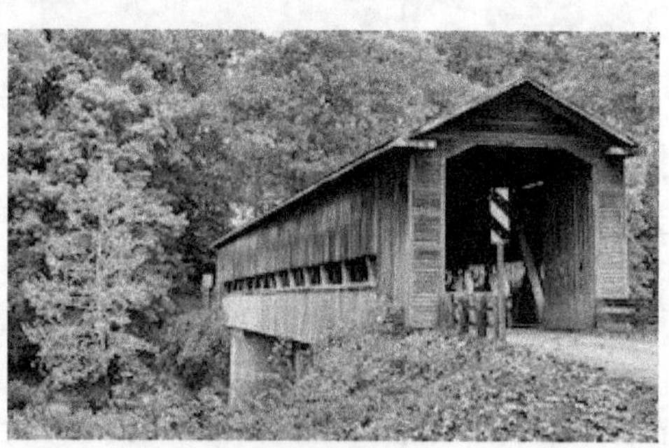

I've probably snapped photos of over a hundred covered bridges and I never seem to tire of them. There has been a concerted effort to preserve them in place, when possible, but some have been moved to protect them. This has been aided by a new competition between states as to who has the most, the best and the most beautiful covered bridges in America. Pennsylvania seems to be the leader in quantity, with 219 still remaining in place. Kentucky was known to have had as many as 700 covered bridges in its history, but only a dozen remain, and, similarly, over 400 were built in New Hampshire with only 54 surviving. Ohio had an amazing 4,000 in its history, but that number has dwindled to just 42, 40 of which I have photographed. The Clint Eastwood-Meryl Streep movie, *The Bridges of Madison County*, in 1995 also served to generate new interest in covered bridges.

As you would expect, the first bridges were made by nature, as fallen trees made a path across a river or stream. The first bridges made by humans were most likely made from logs, planks and stones with little or no support structure. Interestingly the first cable-connecting spans were designed after watching monkeys swing on vines from tree to tree. The first such bridges were constructed in China as early as 206 BC. Expertise continued to improve in China and by 605 AD the oldest surviving stone bridge was built during the Sui Dynasty. Of course, the greatest pre-modern bridge builders were the ancient Romans, the first to use a form of cement in their materials. With the Industrial Revolution came steel, then designs of beam, cantilever, arch, suspension, cable-stayed and truss bridges.

The best thing for tourists is the sheer number of bridges of all sorts everywhere in the country, and in most of the world. Whether you aspire to take the perfect bridge photograph or just enjoy visiting historical structures, there is much to like about bridges, and many to like.

=================

I'll leave the discussion with a particularly appropriate quote from 20th-century architect Santiago Calatrava, who said, *"What I do is the opposite of building walls. I build bridges. A bridge is something that connects instead of separating."*

Acknowledgments

My articles aren't meant to be science lessons and not every source is credited. If you have a question about a fact or figure I mention, please feel free to look it up.

I thoroughly enjoyed searching for quotations to go with each topic. Most quotes were taken from Brainyquote.com.

Most photos were mine, but some royalty-free pics were from Pexels.com, which does not require posting photographer credit. I would, however, highly recommend the site for your personal needs.

I want to thank Andrea Ashley for her professional and often essential proof-reading and editing services on many of my published books, including this one. Anyone who doubts the difficulty of this task needs only to offer to perform it for someone.

Last, I want to thank Gerri Almand for her moral support and graciously writing a couple of paragraphs for my Forward. If you get a chance, her RV-lifestyle books, *The Reluctant RV Wife* and *Home is Where the RV Is*, are amusing and can be helpful glimpses into the full-time RV life.

About the Author

About Me

I am an RV full-timer, living on the road with my wife, Nadyne, and our two Chihuahua-mixes, Rosie and Sadie. I believe I have found a niche in the detective, mystery and crime/thriller genres with several Pat Ruger Mystery Series novels on the market, but also in the RV marketplace, with a several dozen articles posted in travel and RV-industry periodicals and websites, and a lighthearted book published about the RV lifestyle.

I also have several books of poetry and photography on the market and have been a Staff Writer for Poetic Monthly Magazine. My first poems were published when I was just 10 years old when two pieces submitted by a teacher were accepted by a literary magazine. I have since written poetry off and on throughout my life.

Being able to weave mysteries was unexpected but understandable, considering my influences growing up. I have always had a penchant for telling stories and I admired this quality in my uncle, Pat. No, Pat Ruger was not modeled after my uncle... Interestingly, my uncle Pat and his wife, Shirley, also spent several years touring the country in their RV.

Social Media

Like many authors, I have many accounts on social media with which to communicate. You can find many of them on my website at *www.jackhuber.com*.

Here are some of my author accounts:

Patreon.com/jackhuber
Amazon.com/author/jackhuber
Facebook.com/JackHuberAuthor
Twitter.com/huberjack
Linkedin.com/in/jackhuber/

Also, I enjoy receiving email from readers: jack@jackhuber.com